PTP

The ASNT PERSONNEL TRAINING PUBLICATIONS

ULTRASONIC TESTING CLASSROOM TRAINING BOOK

Written for ASNT by

Paul T. Marks
NDT Training Center

The American Society for Nondestructive Testing, Inc.

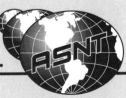

Published by The American Society for Nondestructive Testing, Inc.
1711 Arlingate Lane
Columbus, OH 43228-0518

ASNT exists to create a safer world by promoting the profession and technologies of nondestructive testing.

ISBN-13: 978-1-57117-119-1

Printed in the United States of America

Library of Congress Cataloging-in-Publication Data
Marks, Paul T.
 Ultrasonic testing classroom training book / written for ASNT by Paul T. Marks.
  p. cm. -- (Personnel training publications series)
 Includes bibliographical references and index.
 ISBN-13: 978-1-57117-119-1 (pbk.)
 1. Ultrasonic testing. I. American Society for Nondestructive Testing. II. Title.

TA417.4.M37 2005
620.1'1274--dc22
        2005007026

First printing 03/07
Second printing 08/08
Third printing with revisions 01/10
Fourth printing with revisions 06/11
Fifth printing 08/12

Acknowledgments

A special thank you goes to the following reviewers who helped with this publication:

John Brunk, Honeywell FM&T
Eugene Chemma, ISG Burns Harbor, LLC
John G. Dendy, NDT Training Center
Louis Elliott, Lockheed Martin
Jerry Fulin, Tennessee Gas Pipeline
Amos Holt, Southwest Research Institute
Jim Houf, The American Society for Nondestructive Testing
Scott Huddleston, Huddleston Technical Services
Doron Kishoni, Business Solutions USA
Stephen Lakata, Norfolk Southern Corporation
Don Locke, Karta Technologies, Inc.
Brian MacCracken, Pratt and Whitney
Joe Mackin, International Pipe Inspectors Association
Michael V. McGloin, NDT Enterprises
S. O. McMillan, BAV Quality Assurance
Joseph E. Monroe, Eastern NDT
Robert Plumstead, Testwell Laboratories, Inc.
Mark Pompe, West Penn Non-Destructive Testing, Inc.
Sam Robinson, Sherwin, Inc.
Robert Saunders, Ellwood City Forge
Frank Sattler, Sattler Consultants, Inc.
Simon Senibi, Boeing Phantom Works
Stephen Senne, Senne Technical Services
David A. Stubbs, University of Dayton Research Institute
Ron VanArsdale, Inspection Training and Consulting
Albert M. Wenzig, Jr., Industrial Testing Laboratory Services, LLC

The Publications Review Committee includes:

Chair, Sharon I. Vukelich, University of Dayton Research Institute
Joe Mackin, International Pipe Inspectors Association
Bruce Smith, University of Texas – San Antonio

Ann E. Spence
Educational Materials Editor

Foreword

The American Society for Nondestructive Testing, Inc. (ASNT) has prepared this series of *Personnel Training Publications* to present the major areas in each nondestructive testing method. Each classroom training book in the series is organized to follow the Recommended Training Course Outlines found in *Recommended Practice No. SNT-TC-1A*. The Level I and Level II candidates should use this classroom training book as a preparation tool for nondestructive testing certification. A Level I or Level II may be expected to know additional information based on industry or employer requirements.

Table of Contents

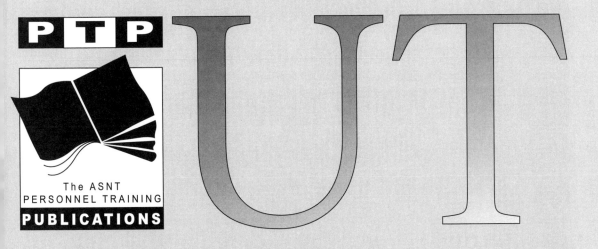

PTP

The ASNT
PERSONNEL TRAINING
PUBLICATIONS

UT

LEVEL I

Chapter 1

Introduction to Ultrasonic Testing

INTRODUCTION

The complexity and expense of today's machines, equipment and tools dictate fabrication and testing procedures that will ensure maximum reliability. To accomplish such reliability, test specifications have been set and test results must meet the criteria established in these specifications. Of the number of nondestructive testing procedures available, ultrasonic testing is one of the most widely used. The test method is regularly used to measure the thickness or to examine the internal structure of a material for possible discontinuities, such as voids and/or cracks.

The purpose of this classroom training book is to provide the fundamental knowledge of ultrasonic testing required by quality assurance and test personnel to enable them to: ascertain that the proper test technique, or combination of techniques, is used to ensure the quality of the finished product; interpret, evaluate and make a sound decision as to the results of the test; and recognize those areas exhibiting doubtful test results that require either retesting or assistance in interpretation and testing.

DEFINITION OF ULTRASONICS

Ultrasonics is the name given to the study and application of sound waves having frequencies higher than those that the human ear can hear. The traditional definition has held that ultrasound begins at 20 000 cycles per second (20 kHz). Compared to that definition, the frequencies used for testing of materials are significantly higher.

Ultrasonic testing frequencies commonly range from 50 000 cycles per second (50 kHz) to 25 000 000 cycles per second (25 MHz). Applications have recently been developed that use frequencies in the range of 400 MHz for testing laminated materials.

Ultrasonic testing uses ultrasonic waves to test materials without destroying them. An ultrasonic test may be used to measure the thickness of a material or to examine the internal structure of a material for possible discontinuities, such as voids and/or cracks.

History of Ultrasonic Testing

For centuries, objects were tested by hitting them with a mallet and listening for a tonal quality difference. Around 1900, railroad workers tested objects by applying kerosene to the object and covering it with a coat of whiting. Then the object was struck with a mallet. In areas where the whiting looked wet, the object was assumed to be cracked. In the early 1940s, Floyd Firestone developed the first pulse echo instrument for detecting deep seated discontinuities. The establishment of basic standards and the first practical immersion testing system is credited to William Hitt and Donald Erdman.

Ultrasonic testing is used to test a variety of both metallic and nonmetallic products, such as welds, forgings, castings, sheet, tubing, plastics (both fiber reinforced and unreinforced) and ceramics. Since ultrasonic testing is capable of economically revealing subsurface discontinuities (variations in material composition) in a variety of dissimilar materials, it is one of the most effective tools available to quality assurance personnel.

Basic Math Review

Most of the math required to understand the physics of ultrasound involves fairly simple equations. The math helps understand the principles of ultrasound in terms of velocity, distance and angles. The following is an example of how the principles and the supporting math are used to explain the characteristics of ultrasound.

Principle

Sound is the mechanical vibration of particles in a material. When a sound wave travels in a material, the particles in the material vibrate around a fixed point at the same frequency as the sound wave. The particles do not travel with the wave, but only react to the energy of the wave. It is the energy of the wave that moves through the material. This concept is illustrated in Figure 1.1.

If the length of a particular sound wave is measured from trough to trough, or from crest to crest, the distance is always the same, as shown in Figure 1.2. This distance is known as the *wavelength*. The time it takes for the wave to travel a distance of one complete wavelength is the same amount of time it takes for the source to execute one complete vibration.

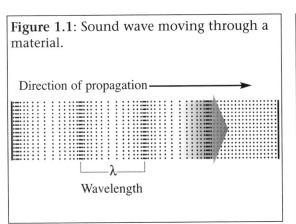

Figure 1.1: Sound wave moving through a material.

Direction of propagation ⟶

Wavelength

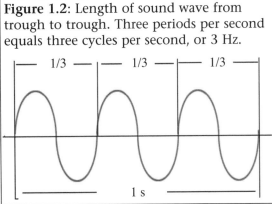

Figure 1.2: Length of sound wave from trough to trough. Three periods per second equals three cycles per second, or 3 Hz.

The velocity of sound *V* is given by Eq. 1.1.

Eq. 1.1 $V = \lambda \times F$

where λ is the wavelength of the wave (most often expressed in millimeters), *V* is the velocity of sound (most often expressed in kilometers) and *F* is the frequency of the wave (most often expressed in megahertz).

QUALIFICATION

It is imperative that personnel responsible for ultrasonic testing are trained and highly qualified with a technical understanding of the test equipment and materials, the test object and the test procedures.

The American Society for Nondestructive Testing (ASNT) has published guidelines for training and qualifying nondestructive testing personnel since 1966. These are known as *Personnel Qualification and Certification in Nondestructive Testing: Recommended Practice No. SNT-TC-1A*. *Recommended Practice No. SNT-TC-1A* describes the responsibilities of nondestructive testing personnel in terms of certification levels.

Levels of Qualification

There are three basic levels of qualification applied to nondestructive testing personnel used by companies that follow *Recommended Practice No. SNT-TC-1A*: Level I, Level II and Level III.

An individual in the process of becoming qualified or certified in Level I ultrasonic testing is considered a trainee. A trainee does not independently conduct tests or interpret, evaluate or report test results of any nondestructive testing method. A trainee works under the direct guidance of certified individuals.

Qualification Requirements for Level I

Level I personnel are qualified to perform the following tasks:

1. Perform specific calibrations, nondestructive tests and evaluations for determining the acceptance or rejection of tested objects in accordance with specific written instructions.
2. Record test results. Normally, the Level I does not have the authority to sign off on the acceptance and completion of the nondestructive test unless specifically trained to do so with clearly written instructions.
3. Perform nondestructive testing job activities in accordance with written instructions or direct supervision from a Level II or Level III technician.

Qualification Requirements for Level II

Level II personnel are qualified to perform the following tasks:

1. Be thoroughly familiar with the scope and limitations of each method for which the individual is certified.
2. Set up and calibrate equipment.
3. Interpret and evaluate results with respect to applicable codes, standards and specifications.
4. Organize and report the results of nondestructive tests.
5. Exercise assigned responsibility for on the job training and guidance of Level I and trainee personnel.

Qualification Requirements for Level III

Level III personnel are qualified to perform the following tasks:

1. Be responsible for nondestructive testing operations to which assigned and for which certified.
2. Develop, qualify and approve procedures; establish and approve nondestructive testing methods and techniques to be used by Level I and II personnel.
3. Interpret and evaluate test results in terms of applicable codes, standards, specifications and procedures.
4. Assist in establishing acceptance criteria where none are available, based on a practical background in applicable materials, fabrication and product technology.
5. Be generally familiar with appropriate nondestructive testing methods other than those for which specifically certified, as demonstrated by passing an ASNT Level III Basic examination.
6. In the methods for which certified, be responsible for, and capable of, training and examination of Level I and Level II personnel for certification in those methods.

Challenges

The major challenge facing nondestructive testing personnel is to learn all that can possibly be learned during the qualification processes. After becoming certified, another challenge involves developing the mindset that there is something else to learn each time the nondestructive testing method is used. There is no substitute for knowledge, and nondestructive testing personnel must be demanding of themselves. The work performed in the nondestructive testing field deserves the very best because of the direct effect of protecting life or endangering life.

CERTIFICATION

It is important to understand the difference between two terms that are often confused within the field of nondestructive testing: *qualification* and *certification*. Qualification is a process that should take place before a person can become certified.

According to *Recommended Practice No. SNT-TC-1A*, the qualification process for any nondestructive testing method should involve the following:

1. Formal training in the fundamental principles and applications of the method.
2. Experience in the application of the method under the guidance of a certified individual (on the job training).
3. Demonstrated ability to pass written and practical (hands on) tests that prove comprehensive understanding of the method and ability to perform actual tests by use of the specific nondestructive testing method.
4. The ability to pass a vision test for visual acuity and color perception.

The actual certification of a person in nondestructive testing to a Level I, Level II or Level III is simply a written testament that the individual has been properly qualified. It should contain the name of the individual being certified, identification of the method and level of certification, the date and the name of the person issuing the certification. Certification is meant to document the actual qualification of the individual.

Correct qualification and certification is extremely important because the process of testing performed by certified nondestructive testing personnel can have a direct impact on the health and safety of every person who will work on, in or in proximity to, the assemblies being tested. Poor work performed by unqualified personnel can cost lives.

Modern fabrication and manufacturing projects challenge the strength and endurance of the joining techniques (such as welding) and the materials of construction. Preventive maintenance activities also present a challenge to nondestructive testing personnel.

The industries that depend on nondestructive testing cannot tolerate testing personnel who are not thoroughly qualified. Too much depends on the judgments made in the work performed every day.

Employee Certification

Training

Training involves an organized program developed to provide test personnel with the knowledge and skill necessary for qualification in a specific area. This is typically performed in a classroom setting where the principles and techniques of the particular test method are reviewed. Online training is also available. The length of training required is stated in the employer's written practice.

Experience

Experience includes work activities accomplished in a particular test method under the supervision of a qualified and/or certified individual in that particular method. This is to include time spent setting up tests, performing calibrations, specific tests and other related activities. Time spent in organized training programs does not count as experience. The length of experience required is stated in the employer's written practice.

Examination

Level I and Level II personnel shall be given written general and specific examinations, a practical examination and a visual examination. The general examination shall cover the basic principles of the applicable method. The specific examination shall cover the procedures, equipment and techniques that the employee will be required to perform in their job assignment. The practical (hands on) examination allows employees to demonstrate their ability to operate the appropriate test equipment and to perform tests using that equipment in accordance with appropriate specifications. Level III personnel must pass written basic, method and specific examinations. Testing requirements are stated in the employer's written practice.

Certification

Certification of nondestructive testing personnel is the responsibility of the employer. Personnel may be certified when they have completed the initial training, experience and examination requirements described in the employer's written practice. The length of certification is stated in the employer's written practice. All applicants shall have documentation that states their qualifications according to the requirements of the written practice before certifications are issued.

Chapter 2

Basic Principles of Acoustics

NATURE OF SOUND WAVES

When a tuning fork is struck, it vibrates and produces sound waves by compressing the air. These waves travel through air to the ear of the listener, as shown in Figure 2.1. The tuning fork vibrations soon die out and no longer produce waves.

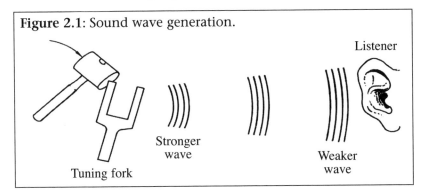

Figure 2.1: Sound wave generation.

Similarly, in ultrasonic testing a short pulse of electrical current excites a transducer (crystal) that vibrates, as did the tuning fork. The sound beam from the transducer then travels through a couplant, which may be water or oil, to the front surface of the test object. Figure 2.2 shows the transducer in contact with the test object and the sound beam pulses traveling through the test object.

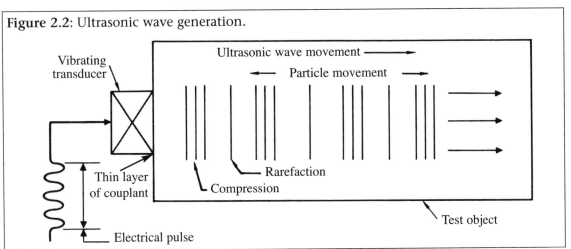

Figure 2.2: Ultrasonic wave generation.

MODES OF SOUND WAVE GENERATION

In general, all types of sound waves travel through solid matter. As a matter of fact, a solid is a much better carrier of sound energy than air because of its rigidity and density. Even a liquid, due to its greater density, is a more efficient carrier of sonic energy than air.

The sound waves that are used in ultrasonic testing are differentiated mainly by the type of vibrational motion set off within the particle structures that lie within the path of a given wave form. There are longitudinal waves, also known as *compression waves*, where the particles of the matter vibrate back and forth in the same direction as the motion of the sound wave. There are shear waves, also known as *transverse waves*, where the particles vibrate back and forth in a direction that is at right angles to the motion of the wave.

It is also possible to produce sound waves that travel along the free boundary (surface) of a solid. These are referred to as *surface waves* (or *Rayleigh waves*) because they penetrate the material to a depth of only a few wavelengths and cause an undulating movement of that surface, much like a wave caused by a pebble dropped into a pond. Finally, a fourth wave mode is the Lamb wave, also known also as *plate wave*.

Propagation of Sound Energy

All materials are made of atoms linked by electromagnetic forces. Solid test objects usually have dense atomic structure compared to liquid and air, and also have degrees of resiliency that allow vibratory movement of the particles within a certain range.

Imagine a lattice work structure where balls (atoms) are interconnected by springs (electromagnetic forces), as was shown in Figure 1.1. If the side of this lattice structure is struck, the first column of atoms exerts a force on the second column, which in turn exerts a force on the third column, and so on, in sequence. After each column of atoms is forced to move, it rebounds back in the other direction. This particle motion produces a wave movement in the direction away from the point where the energy was introduced. In the case shown in Figure 2.3, the particle movement would be back and forth in a direction that is parallel to the direction of the energy travel within the solid. Relating to sound, this type of sound wave motion is known as the *longitudinal* (or *compression*) *wave mode*.

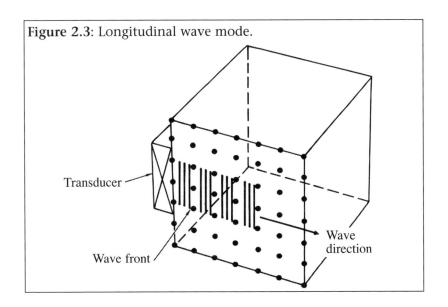

Figure 2.3: Longitudinal wave mode.

Transducer

Wave front

Wave direction

COMPARISON OF WAVE MODES

Longitudinal Wave Mode

Figure 2.4 shows two transducers generating ultrasonic waves in the same test object. Note that the transducer on the left is producing longitudinal waves. The back and forth vibration of particles, parallel to the direction of wave travel, promotes efficient energy transfer. Longitudinal waves can be transmitted through solids, liquids and even gases, such as air. This is not true of the other modes of sound energy. Shear, surface and plate waves can be transmitted only within a solid material.

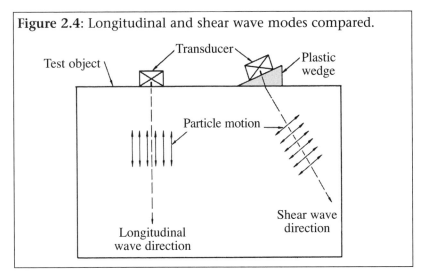

Figure 2.4: Longitudinal and shear wave modes compared.

Test object

Transducer

Plastic wedge

Particle motion

Longitudinal wave direction

Shear wave direction

Shear Wave Mode

In Figure 2.4, the transducer on the right is producing a different kind of wave. This is called a *shear wave* because the particle movement direction is at right angles to the wave movement direction, otherwise referred to as the *direction of propagation*. The velocity of shear waves through a material is about half that of the longitudinal wave. Note also that the right hand transducer is mounted on a plastic wedge so that the ultrasonic waves generated by the crystal enter the material at a specific angle. This specific angle, plus the velocity of the wave within the material, determines the angle of sound propagation.

Confusion may be encountered when angle beam transducers, designed to produce a specific refracted angle in one kind of material, are applied to other materials with different acoustic velocities. A transducer designed to produce a shear wave beam at 45° in steel, for example, will produce a shear wave beam at 43° in aluminum or 30° in copper.

Rayleigh Wave Mode

A third wave type is confined to a thin layer of particles on the free boundary of a solid material. Rayleigh waves travel over the surface of a solid and bear a rough resemblance to waves produced by a pebble dropped onto the surface of a pond. They were named for Lord Rayleigh because of his research on earthquakes, and his identification of the rolling wave as the principal component of the energy waves that travel along the surface of the Earth.

These Rayleigh waves are otherwise known as *surface waves*, and are used extensively in ultrasonic testing applications today. They travel at a velocity of 117 200 in. (297 688 cm) per second in steel compared to the shear wave velocity of 128 000 in. (325 120 cm) per second. Thus, Rayleigh waves travel in steel at 91.6% the velocity of shear waves, or 8.4% less. As shown in

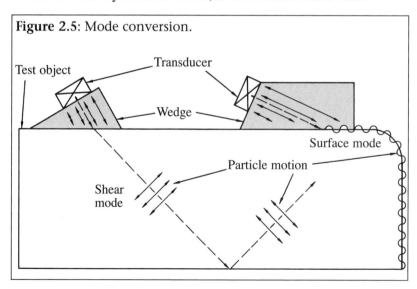

Figure 2.5: Mode conversion.

Test object

Transducer

Wedge

Surface mode

Particle motion

Shear
mode

Figure 2.5, when a transducer is mounted on a steeply angled plastic wedge, the longitudinal beam in the wedge strikes the test surface at a high angle, producing a surface wave in the test object. As shown, a surface wave can travel around a curve. Reflection of the surface wave occurs only at a sharp corner or at a discontinuity. Figure 2.6 illustrates the particle motion within a Rayleigh wave beam.

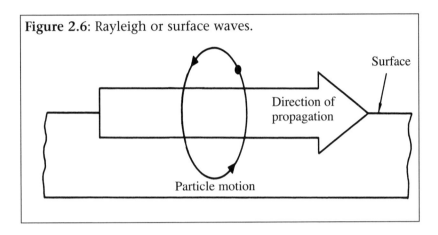

Figure 2.6: Rayleigh or surface waves.

Lamb Waves

If a surface wave is introduced into a material that has a thickness equal to three wavelengths or less of the ultrasound, a different kind of wave results. The material begins to vibrate as a plate because the wave encompasses the entire thickness of the material. When this occurs, the normal rules for wave velocity cease to apply. The velocity is no longer solely dependent on the type of material and the type of wave. Instead, a wave velocity is produced that is influenced by the frequency of the wave, in addition to the angle of incidence and the type of material. The theory describing Lamb waves was developed by Horace Lamb in 1916, and therefore carries his name.

Lamb Wave Types

There are two general types of Lamb (or plate) waves depending on the way the particles in the material move as the wave moves along the plate. Both types are shown in Figure 2.7.

Lamb Wave Modes

Each type of Lamb wave has an infinite number of modes that the wave may attain. These modes are dependent on the three factors: the frequency of the wave, the angle of incidence and the material. These modes are differentiated by the manner in which the particles in the material are moving. Figure 2.7 illustrates the first mode, whereas Figure 2.8 illustrates the second and third modes.

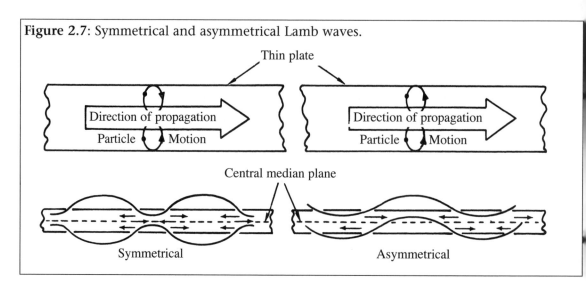

Figure 2.7: Symmetrical and asymmetrical Lamb waves.

Thin plate

Direction of propagation

Particle Motion

Direction of propagation

Particle Motion

Central median plane

Symmetrical

Asymmetrical

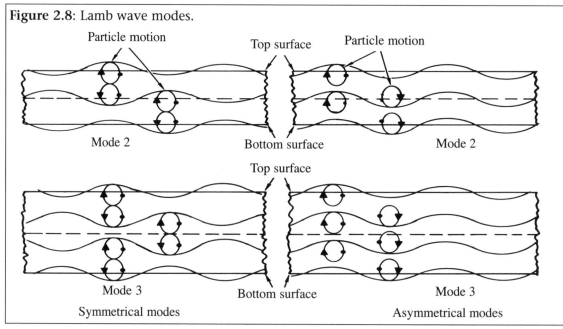

Figure 2.8: Lamb wave modes.

Particle motion

Top surface

Particle motion

Mode 2

Bottom surface

Mode 2

Top surface

Mode 3

Bottom surface

Mode 3

Symmetrical modes

Asymmetrical modes

The ability of Lamb waves to flow in thin plates makes them applicable to a wide variety of problems requiring the detection of subsurface discontinuities. The first modes do not reveal subsurface discontinuities because their energy is contained close to the surface of the medium, as with Rayleigh waves. Where it is desirable that energy travels a considerable distance along the plate, or where detection of subsurface discontinuities is required, adjustments in applied frequency can produce velocities near that of the longitudinal mode. These modes are useful for immersion testing of thin walled tubing and plates for internal discontinuities or grain size determinations and testing of welds in thin plates and tubes.

Table 2.1 lists the modes produced by various incident angles when transmitting a 5 MHz ultrasonic beam into a 0.13 cm (0.05 in.) thick aluminum plate.

Table 2.1: Lamb wave modes in aluminum.	
Incident Angle	**Mode Produced**
33°	First asymmetrical
31°	First symmetrical
25.6°	Second asymmetrical
19.6°	Second symmetrical
14.7°	Third asymmetrical
12.6°	Third symmetrical
7.8°	Fourth symmetrical

Velocity, Frequency and Wavelength

Ultrasonic wave vibrations possess properties very similar to those of light waves. For example, they may be reflected, focused and refracted. The high frequency particle vibrations of sound waves are propagated in homogeneous solid objects in the same manner as a directed light beam might pass through clear air. Sound beams are reflected (partially or totally) at any surface acting as a boundary between the object and a gas, liquid or another type of solid. As with echo sounding in sonar applications, the ultrasonic pulses reflect from discontinuities and enable detection and location of the interface.

Attenuation of Sound Waves

High frequency ultrasonic waves passing through a material are reduced in power, or attenuated, by several mechanisms including reflection and scattering of the beams at the grain boundaries within the material and friction losses. The reflection and scattering losses are proportional to the grain volume in the material and the wavelength of the beam. Scattering losses are greatest where the wavelength is less than one third of the grain size. As the frequency is lowered and the wavelength becomes greater than the grain size, attenuation is caused only by damping of the wave. In damping losses, wave energy is lost through heat caused by friction of the vibrating particles.

Acoustical Impedance

Acoustical impedance is the resistance of a medium to the passage of sound waves. The impedance Z of any material may be computed by multiplying the density of the material ρ by the velocity of sound V through the material.

Eq. 2.1 $Z = \rho V$

Air has a very low impedance to ultrasonic waves because it is low in density (p) and slow in velocity (V). The impedance of water is higher than the impedance of air, and solids such as aluminum and steel have even higher impedances.

Impedance Ratio

When a transducer is used to transmit an ultrasonic wave into a material, only part of the wave energy is transmitted; the rest is reflected from the surface of the material. Also, some amount of ultrasonic energy is reflected at the interface between two different materials as a sound beam passes from one to the other. How much of the sound beam is reflected depends on a factor called *acoustical impedance ratio*.

The acoustical impedance ratio between two materials is simply the acoustical impedance of one material divided by the acoustical impedance of the other material. When an ultrasonic beam is passing from material A into material B, the impedance ratio is the impedance of the second material divided by the impedance of the first material. The higher the ratio, the more of the original energy will be reflected.

Since air has a very small impedance, the impedance ratio between air and any liquid or solid material is very high, therefore most, if not all, of the sound beam will be reflected at any interface between air and any other material.

A high impedance ratio is often called an *impedance mismatch*. If the impedance ratio, for example, was 5:1, the impedance mismatch would be 5:1. Whereas the impedance ratio for air-to-metal is about 115 000:1 (virtually 100% reflection), the impedance ratio for a liquid-to-metal interface is lower. For example, the acoustic impedance values of water and steel are 0.148 and 4.616, respectively, making the impedance ratio about 31:1. Reflection may be calculated by using the following formula:

Eq. 2.2
$$R = \frac{(Z_2 - Z_1)^2}{(Z_2 + Z_1)^2}$$

where Z_1 is the impedance value of the first material and Z_2 that of the second. Inserting the above values, a value of 88% reflection at the water-to-steel interface is obtained:

$$R = \frac{(4.616 - 0.148)^2}{(4.616 + 0.148)^2} = \frac{4.468^2}{4.764^2} = \frac{19.963}{22.696} = 0.88$$

REFLECTION

In many ways, a beam of ultrasonic waves acts in the same way as a beam of light waves. For example, when they strike an interrupting test object, some or most of the sound beam energy is reflected. These

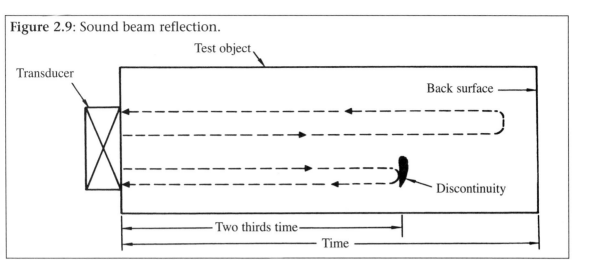

Figure 2.9: Sound beam reflection.

reflections may then be picked up by a second, or, in many cases, by the same transducer.

Ultrasonic testing does not give direct information about the exact nature of the discontinuity. This is deduced from several factors, the most important being knowledge of the test object's material and its construction. Ultrasonic waves are reflected from both the discontinuity and the back surface of the test object as echoes. The echo from the discontinuity is received before the back surface reflection is received. Figure 2.9 shows a situation where the time required for the sound beam to travel through the test object to the discontinuity and back is only two thirds of the time required for the sound beam to reach to the back surface and return. This time differential indicates that the discontinuity is located two thirds of the distance to the back surface.

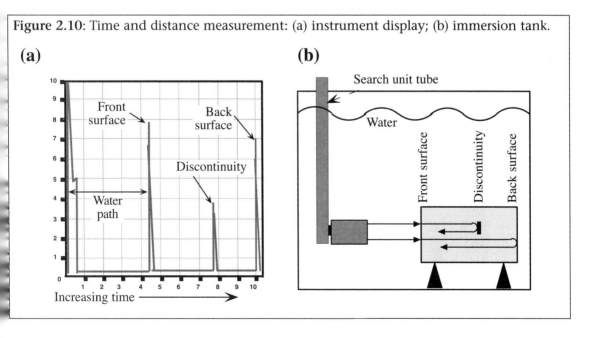

Figure 2.10: Time and distance measurement: (a) instrument display; (b) immersion tank.

The distance that the sound beam travels to a reflecting surface can be measured on the display screen of the ultrasonic instrument, as shown in Figure 2.10. The initial pulse and the echo from the front surface of the test object produce the first two sharp indications that rise from the base line of the instrument display screen. The distance between these two indications is proportional to the distance between the transducer and the front surface.

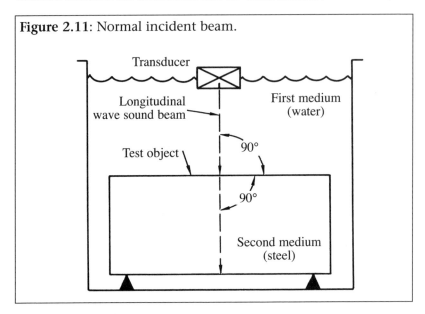

Figure 2.11: Normal incident beam.

REFRACTION AND MODE CONVERSION

Refraction and mode conversion of the ultrasonic beam as it passes at an angle from one material to another is comparable to the refraction of light beams when passing from one medium to another.

Figure 2.11 shows a transducer inducing a longitudinal sound beam into water. The water transmits the beam to the test object. When the longitudinal wave sound beam is incident to the surface of the test object in the perpendicular direction, the beam is transmitted through the first and second medium as a 100% longitudinal beam and no refraction occurs.

Mixed Mode Conversion
As shown in Figure 2.12, as the incident angle is changed from the initial 90° position, refraction and mode conversion occur. The original longitudinal beam is transmitted in the second medium as varying percentages of both longitudinal and shear wave beams. As shown, the refracted angle for the longitudinal wave beam is four times the incident angle, and the shear wave beam angle is a little more than twice the incident angle. If the incident angle is rotated further, the refraction angles of the longitudinal wave and the shear

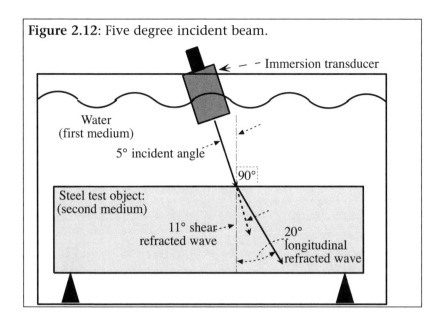

Figure 2.12: Five degree incident beam.

Immersion transducer

Water
(first medium)

5° incident angle

90°

Steel test object:
(second medium)

11° shear
refracted wave

20°
longitudinal
refracted wave

wave increase. The value of each refracted beam varies in the test object as the angle of incidence in the first medium is changed.

Refraction and mode conversion occur because the speed of the longitudinal wave changes when the beam enters the second medium. The velocity of the shear wave is about half that of the longitudinal wave, so the change in angel in approximately one-half as much. As the incident angle is rotated further, the refracted angle of each wave mode increases until the longitudinal wave reaches a refraction angle of 90°. This point can be calculated by use of Snell's law. It is identified as the first critical angle, and refers to the incident angle that produces the 90° refraction of the longitudinal wave.

SNELL'S LAW AND CRITICAL ANGLES

In angle beam testing, when the ultrasonic velocities in the liquid (used in immersion testing) or the wedge material (used in contact testing) are different from the ultrasonic velocity in the test object, the longitudinal beam passing through the wedge or couplant is refracted when the sound beam enters the test object. Incident or refracted angles may be computed by an equation known as *Snell's law*.

Snell's Law Calculations

Snell's law states that the sine of the angle of incidence in the first medium is to the sine of the angle of refraction in the second medium as the velocity of sound in the first medium is to the velocity of sound in the second medium. Snell's law is expressed mathematically in Eq. 2.3.

Eq. 2.3 $\dfrac{\sin \theta_I}{\sin \theta_R} = \dfrac{V_I}{V_R}$

where θ_I is the incident angle from normal of the beam in the liquid or wedge, θ_R is the angle of the refracted beam in the test material, V_I is the velocity of incident beam in the liquid or wedge and V_R is the velocity of refracted beam in the test object.

The calculations for determining angles of incidence or refraction require trigonometric tables. The sine (sin) ratios are given in decimal fractions. Velocities are often given in centimeters per microsecond (cm/μs). To convert from units of cm/μs to units of (cm/s) × 10⁵, move the decimal one place to the right. Multiply in./s by 2.54 to obtain cm/s. Snell's law can be used to determine angular relationships between media for both longitudinal and shear waves.

Figure 2.13: Calculation of refracted angle for longitudinal waves and shear waves.

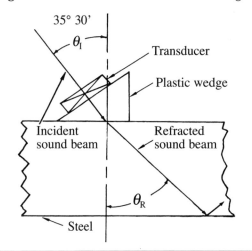

Snell's law: $\dfrac{\sin\theta_I}{\sin\theta_R} = \dfrac{V_I}{V_R}$

Given:
V_I (for longitudinal waves in plastic)
= 0.267 cm/μs
V_R (for longitudinal waves in steel)
= 0.585 cm/μs
V_R (for shear waves in steel)
= 0.323 cm/μs
$\sin\theta_I = 35°\ 30' = 0.5807$ from
trigonometric function tables

Solution of Problem for Longitudinal Waves	**Solution of Problem for Shear Waves**
Substitute values in the equation for Snell's law	Substitute values in the equation for Snell's law

Longitudinal Waves:

$$\frac{0.5807}{\sin\theta_R} = \frac{0.267}{0.585}$$

$$\sin\theta_R = \frac{0.585(0.5807)}{0.267}$$

$$\sin\theta_R = 1.2723$$

Since $\sin\theta_R$ is greater than 1, all longitudinal waves are reflected

Shear Waves:

$$\frac{0.5807}{\sin\theta_R} = \frac{0.267}{0.323}$$

$$\sin\theta_R = \frac{0.323(0.5807)}{0.267}$$

$$\sin\theta_R = 0.7024$$

$$\theta_R = 44°\ 37' \text{ from trigonometric sine function } 0.70236.$$

Answer: No longitudinal wave can exist in the steel and the angle of refraction of the shear wave is 44° 37'.

Typical Problem Solving Method

Figure 2.13 shows a contact transducer mounted at an incident angle of 35° 30' on a plastic wedge. The angle of the refracted beam may be calculated with the formula for Snell's law because the incident angle and the velocity of the sound beam in the first and second medium are known. In this case, only shear waves are produced in the steel, as the incident angle is in the region between the first and second critical angles.

CRITICAL ANGLES OF REFRACTION

Sound beams passing through a medium such as water or plastic are refracted when entering a second medium at an incident angle. For small incident beam angles, sound beams are refracted and subjected to mode conversion, resulting in a combination of shear and longitudinal waves. The region between normal incidence and the first critical angle is not as useful for ultrasonic testing as is the region beyond the first critical angle where only shear waves are produced. The presence of two beams results in confusing signals.

First Critical Angle

As the angle of incidence is increased, the first critical angle is reached when the refracted longitudinal beam angle reaches 90°. At this point, only shear waves exist in the second medium. When selecting a contact shear wave angle beam transducer, or when adjusting an immersed transducer at an incident angle to produce shear waves, two conditions are considered.

First, the refracted longitudinal wave must be totally reflected (its angle of refraction must be 90° or greater) so that the penetrating beam is limited to shear waves only. Second, the refracted shear wave must enter the test object in accordance with the requirements of the test standard. In the immersion method of testing, the first critical angle is calculated to ensure that the sound beam enters the test material at the desired angle.

As the incident angle is increased further, the second critical angle is reached when the refracted shear beam angle reaches 90°. At this point, all shear waves are reflected and, in the case of contact testing with the test object in an air medium, surface waves are produced. In immersion testing, the liquid medium dampens the production of surface waves to a large degree, but it should be noted that surface waves have been produced in experimental tests on immersed test objects.

Calculation of Critical Angles

If the sound beam velocities for the incident wave and for the refracted wave are known (V_I and V_R), either critical angle may be calculated with Snell's law using the sine of 90°. The sin (90°) = 1. Thus, to compute the first critical angle in the case of the contact

transducer mounted on a plastic wedge for testing steel, Eq. 2.4
should be used.

Eq. 2.4 $\quad \dfrac{\sin \theta_I}{\sin \theta_R} = \dfrac{V_I}{V_R \ (longitudinal\ wave)}$

$$\frac{\sin \theta_I}{\sin 90°} = \frac{0.267\,\text{cm}/\mu s}{0.585\,\text{cm}/\mu s} = \frac{\sin \theta_I}{1} = 0.45641$$

Divide V_R into $V_I = 0.45641 = 27° \ 9'$ for first critical angle. If the
second critical angle is desired, V_R is the sound beam velocity for a
shear wave in steel: 0.323 cm/μs. V_R is again divided into
$V_I = 0.82662 = 55° \ 45'$ for the second critical angle.

Table 2.2: Critical angles in immersion testing. First medium is H_2O (V = 0.149 cm/μs).

Test Material	First Critical Angle	Second Critical Angle	Velocity (cm/μs)	
			Longitudinal	Shear
Beryllium	7°	10°	1.280	0.871
Aluminum 17ST	14°	29°	0.625	0.310
Steel	15°	27°	0.585	0.323
Stainless 302	15°	29°	0.566	0.312
Tungsten	17°	31°	0.518	0.287
Uranium	26°	51°	0.338	0.193

Table 2.3: Critical angles in contact testing. First medium is plastic (V = 0.267 cm/μs).

Test Material	First Critical Angle	Second Critical Angle	Velocity (cm/μs)	
			Longitudinal	Shear
Beryllium	12°	18°	1.280	0.871
Aluminum 17ST	25°	59°	0.625	0.310
Steel	27°	56°	0.585	0.323
Stainless 302	28°	59°	0.566	0.312
Tungsten	31°	68°	0.518	0.287
Uranium	52°	–	0.338	0.193

Table 2.2 lists approximate critical angles for various test
materials when water is used as the first medium ($V_I = 0.149$ cm/μs).
Table 2.3 lists approximate critical angles for the same test materials
when a plastic wedge is used as the first medium ($V_I = 0.267$ cm/μs).

Note that uranium does not have a second critical angle in this
case. This is because the shear wave velocity in uranium is less than
the longitudinal wave velocity in plastic. Essentially, this situation
means that the incident angle would have to be greater than 90° to
obtain a 90° refraction of the beam in uranium. An incident angle
greater than 90° is physically impossible.

Sound Beam Patterns

In ultrasonic testing, the ultrasonic beam is generally considered to be a straight sided projection of the face of the transducer. In reality, the beam is not straight sided or even energy consistent along the beam centerline. If the beam intensity is measured at various distances from the transducer, two distinct zones are found, as shown on Figure 2.14. These zones are known as the *near field*, or *Fresnel zone*, and the *far field*, or *Fraunhofer zone*. More information on near fields and far fields is found in Chapter 4.

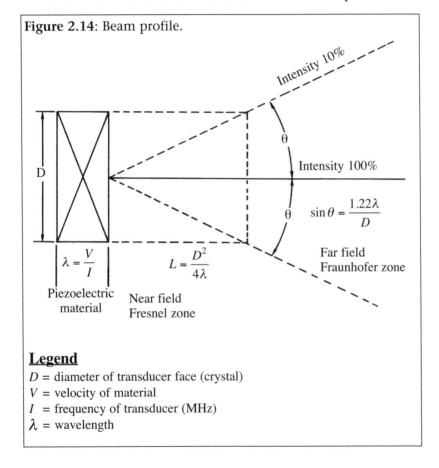

Figure 2.14: Beam profile.

Intensity 10%

θ

Intensity 100%

$\sin \theta = \dfrac{1.22\lambda}{D}$

θ

Far field
Fraunhofer zone

$\lambda = \dfrac{V}{I}$

$L = \dfrac{D^2}{4\lambda}$

Piezoelectric material

Near field
Fresnel zone

D

Legend
D = diameter of transducer face (crystal)
V = velocity of material
I = frequency of transducer (MHz)
λ = wavelength

Chapter 3

Equipment

INTRODUCTION

This chapter covers the more commonly used ultrasonic testing equipment. The manufacturers' manuals, in most cases, provide operation and maintenance instructions for the units, a review of theory and other more specific information. Manufacturers' recommendations supersede this chapter in the event of conflicting information.

Figure 3.1 depicts training in the use of a portable ultrasonic discontinuity detector. This type of unit, and others that are more elaborate, are discussed in this chapter.

Figure 3.1: Ultrasonic testing trainee using a discontinuity detector.

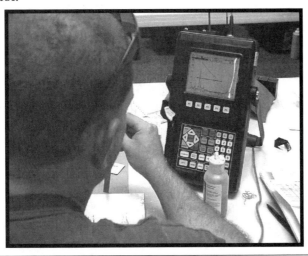

PULSE ECHO INSTRUMENTATION

Ultrasonic testing systems are referred to as being one of three types: A-scan, B-scan or C-scan. In fact, use of the terms relates to the format that is displayed on the screen of the ultrasonic instrument used for a given test. Whether A, B or C-scan, they are, for the most part, dependent on the same basic electronic components. Typical ultrasonic instruments are designed to produce outgoing electronic pulses and to amplify returning echoes from test materials. The essential differences lie in how the incoming information is represented on a display.

A-Scan Equipment

The A-scan system is a signal presentation method that displays the returned signals from the test material on the display screen, as shown in Figure 3.2. The horizontal base line on the screen indicates elapsed time (from left to right). The vertical deflection shows signal amplitudes that allow the technician to gage relative size of the reflector.

Figure 3.2: A-scan presentation.

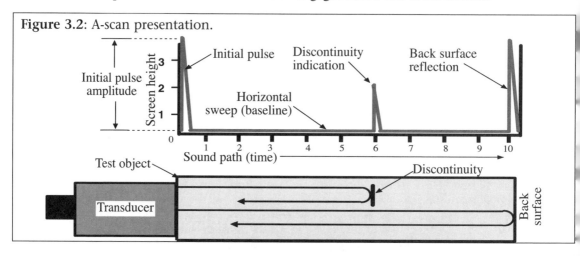

In Figures 3.3 and 3.4, a signal results when the transducer is coupled to a 2.5 cm (1 in.) thick mild steel test block (Figure 3.3). In Figure 3.4, a signal is produced when the same transducer is placed on a 1.9 cm (0.75 in.) test block made of the same material. Notice that the back surface reflections have changed positions. The shorter distance to the 1.9 cm (0.75 in.) reflector is closer to the left side of the display screen and is accurately representing the change in distance between the two reflecting surfaces.

Figure 3.3: Resulting signal when a transducer is coupled to a 2.5 cm (1 in.) thick mild steel test block.

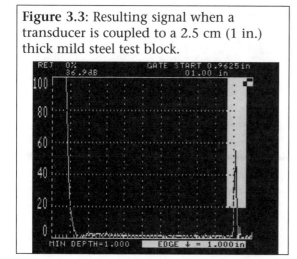

Figure 3.4: Signal is produced when the same transducer shown in Figure 3.3 is placed on a 1.9 cm (0.75 in.) test block made of the same material.

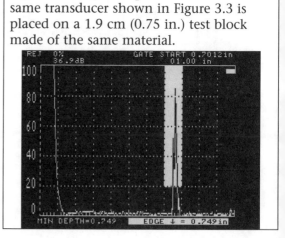

Also notice that the amplitude of the more distant reflector (Figure 3.3) is less than that of the reflector at 1.9 cm (0.75 in.) (Figure 3.4). The increased distance to the more distant surface caused a reduction in amplitude of that signal due to attenuation of the sound energy.

Distance and amplitude information gathered by use of A-scan applications enable the ultrasonic technician to view objective evidence of the conditions encountered within the test object.

B-Scan Equipment

B-scan representation produces a two-dimensional view of the cross-sectional plane through the test object. It is typically used in applications such as corrosion monitoring and lamination detection in metals and composites. The B-scan display produces a view of the test material that looks as if it was cut through and turned on its side. This shows, in cross-section, whatever internal reflectors or opposite surface conditions exist.

Figures 3.5 and 3.6 show an example of a B-scan presentation performed by use of the same instrument used to produce the A-scans shown in Figures 3.3 and 3.4. Manufacturers of most discontinuity detectors provide a B-scan component to users who want the benefit of using the same unit for A and B-scan applications.

Figure 3.5 represents the four steps of a 2.5 cm (1 in.) step wedge, with 1.9, 1.3 and 0.6 cm (0.75, 0.5 and 0.25 in.) steps displayed as a percentage of 2.5 cm (1 in.).

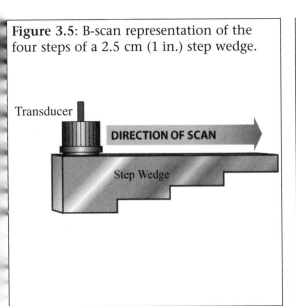

Figure 3.5: B-scan representation of the four steps of a 2.5 cm (1 in.) step wedge.

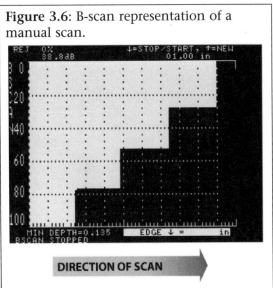

Figure 3.6: B-scan representation of a manual scan.

B-scan equipment provides opportunity for real time visualization of the material condition as it is tested. Figure 3.7 illustrates a B-scan display of internal discontinuities lying under the scanning path of an ultrasonic transducer.

Figure 3.7: B-scan display of internal discontinuities lying under the scanning path of an ultrasonic transducer.

Discontinuities

Front surface

Thickness of test object

Back surface

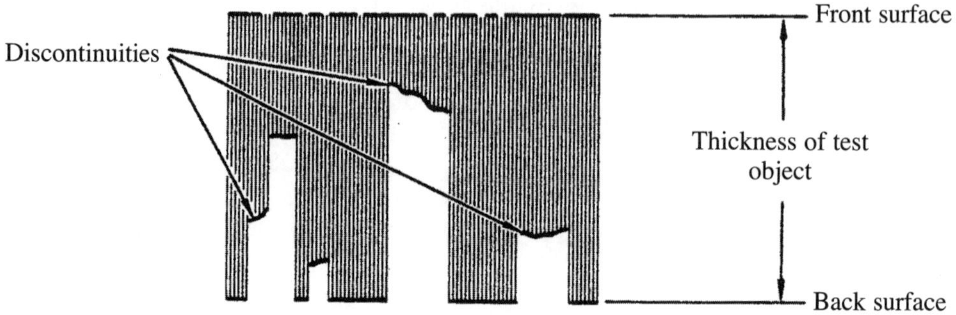

C-Scan Equipment

Another common display of ultrasonic testing data uses a plan view (looking down on the test object) called a *C-scan*. In this approach, the transducer is scanned in a regular pattern over an area of interest, usually using an automatic mechanical positioning device. The received signals are converted to variations in color or grayscale density.

Created from A-scan data, the plan view of the test object is generated using signal criteria based on pulse height and time of arrival to determine color or grayscale density at each X/Y location. This is like the floor plan of a house in that the vertical and horizontal directions represent the area over which the transducer was scanned.

The resulting patterns correlate with the size and shape of the reflecting surfaces within the test object, and are intuitively easy to interpret, like X-ray images. Figure 3.8 represents a C-scan of a test object. The images show the shapes and plan positions of the reflectors.

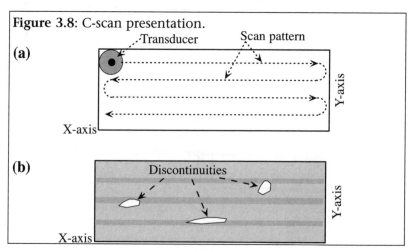

Figure 3.8: C-scan presentation.

(a) Transducer   Scan pattern
Y-axis
X-axis

(b) Discontinuities
Y-axis
X-axis

The major advantage of the C-scan representation is the understandable display of information related to reflector shape and position that is not as readily interpreted when looking at an A-scan or B-scan display.

PULSE ECHO INSTRUMENTATION ELECTRONICS

All makes of pulse echo equipment have similar electronic circuitry and provide basic common functions. Names of the various circuits vary from one instrument to another according to the manufacturer, however each unit must provide certain essentials. The block diagram in Figure 3.9 illustrates these.

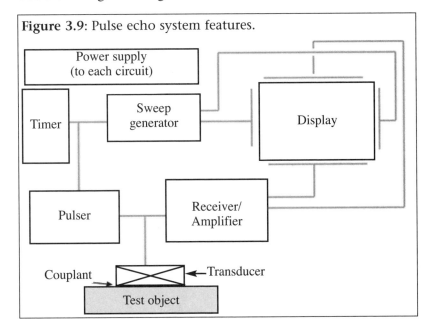

Figure 3.9: Pulse echo system features.

Power Supply

The power supply is usually controlled by an on/off switch and a fuse. After turning the power on, there are certain time delay devices that protect circuit elements during instrument warm up. Circuits for supplying current for all basic functions of the instrument constitute the power supply. Electrical power is served from line supply or, as in the case of portables, from a battery contained in the unit.

Transducer

A transducer is a device that converts energy from one form to another. The ultrasonic transducer consists of a thin piezoelectric disk, sometimes called an *element* or *crystal*, and its holder. The disk converts electrical energy to ultrasonic energy and introduces vibrations into the test object. It also receives reflected ultrasonic vibrations from within the test object and converts them into electrical signals for amplification and display. An in depth review of transducers is found in Chapter 4.

Pulser/Receiver

The pulser, or pulse generator, is the source of short high energy bursts of electrical energy (triggered by the timer) that are applied to the transducer. Return pulses from the test object are received by the transducer, sent to the receiver, amplified and routed to the display unit.

Display and Timer

In modern ultrasonic testing devices, flat panel display screens have replaced the oscilloscope cathode ray tubes (CRT) that had been used in the ultrasonic devices manufactured up to the early 1990s. The displays, whether flat panel or cathode ray tubes of the older analog units, are integrated with a sweep generator and the controls required to provide a visual image of the signals received from the test object. The timer is the source of all timing signals to the pulser, and is sometimes referred to as the *rate generator* or *clock*.

CONTROL FUNCTIONS

Controls are provided for the various circuits of the instrument, such as power supply, pulser, receiver, timer and display. The nomenclature used in the following description of the controls may vary from one type of unit to another. Figure 3.10 illustrates the instrument controls.

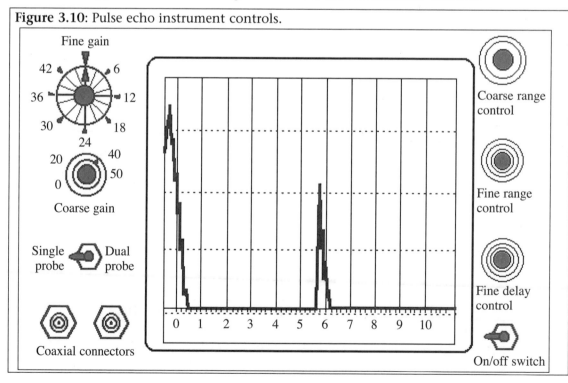

Figure 3.10: Pulse echo instrument controls.

Instrument Gain Controls

Instrument gain controls connect to the amplifier and adjust the amount of amplification that incoming signals from the transducer receive before the screen display is made.

Probe Mode Control

This switch determines if the instrument will drive and display the activity of one transducer or two. When switched to single probe mode, the instrument will send and receive short bursts of electrical energy through a coaxial cable to a single transducer.

When switched to dual probe mode, the instrument directs outbound electrical bursts through the coaxial connector toward one transducer tasked for sending ultrasonic waves into the test object. Inbound signals from the material are received by a separate transducer connected to the other coaxial connector. The result of this setting would be a through transmission or dual probe test, where the sending transducer is isolated from the receiving transducer.

Coarse Range, Fine Range and Delay Controls

These controls serve as a means of causing the instrument screen to adjust the display along the horizontal axis. This display axis usually shows the time, distance or depth of ultrasonic travel in the test object. The coarse range and fine range controls are sometimes called *material calibration* or *material velocity controls*, depending on the manufacturer of the instrument. In fact, these controls allow the technician to perform a basic part of the standardization/ calibration of the instrument.

Coarse range and fine range controls allow for the precise screen placement of signals from known reference distances within standardization blocks. By use of these controls, as well as the delay control, signals from known distances are placed in their correct position on the display screen. This enables the screen to represent the appropriate distance that will allow for complete through dimension testing. By use of standardization blocks made of material like that to be tested, the instrument screen can be set to represent 2.5, 13, 25 cm (1, 5, 10 in.) or more of sound travel within a test object.

Keypad Instrumentation

In addition to the basic controls shown in Figure 3.10, more recently manufactured instruments make use of menu sections that are adjusted from push button keypads instead of knobs and toggle switches. Figure 3.11 illustrates such a keypad that is accessed from the front panel of the instrument. The keypads and menus allow for the adjustment of all functions required for the standardization of the instrument in preparation for the actual test.

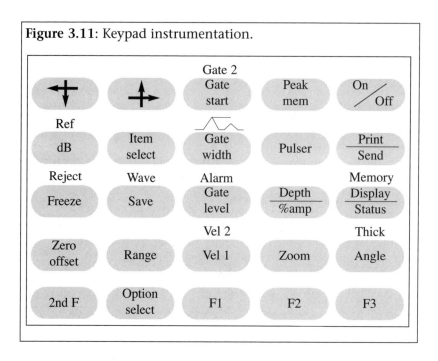

Figure 3.11: Keypad instrumentation.

The following sections refer to Figure 3.11 to discuss various functions of the ultrasonic instrument and the keypad access used by technicians for ultrasonic testing setup.

On/Off Control

The on/off control admits (or stops) the flow of power to the unit's components, enabling (or stopping) operation.

Display/Status Control

The display/status control allows the technician to switch between views of the display screen. For example, the screen could display the A-scan, the instrument settings or a combination of both shown on a so-called *split screen*, as shown in Figure 3.12. Figure 3.12b shows what the technician sees after pressing the display/status button a second time.

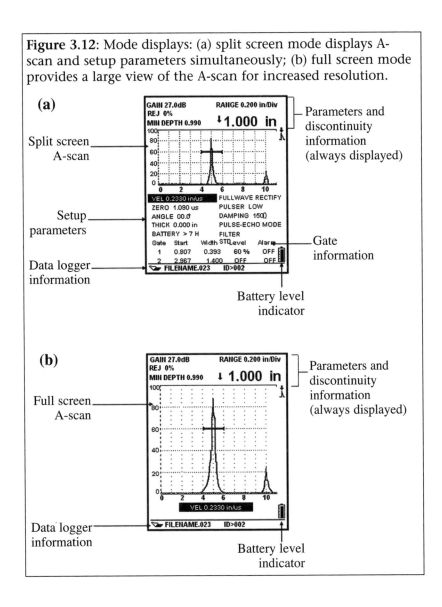

Figure 3.12: Mode displays: (a) split screen mode displays A-scan and setup parameters simultaneously; (b) full screen mode provides a large view of the A-scan for increased resolution.

Gain Control

The gain key controls the amplifier circuit. It does not have any influence over outbound pulses, but has everything to do with signals returning from the test material.

The gain, or system sensitivity, in modern ultrasonic instruments may exceed 100 dB, and is adjustable in increments as small as 0.1 dB. To use the gain control in Figure 3.11, the technician would simply press the decibel key ("dB"), and then the so-called *slewing key*, shown in Figure 3.13.

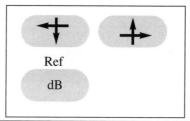

Figure 3.13: Press decibel and slewing keys to adjust system sensitivity.

Ref

dB

Reject Control

The purpose of the reject control is to eliminate unwanted, low level A-scan signals. It is particularly useful in the inspection of typically coarse grained castings. This control also works on the amplifier circuit.

Zero Offset Control

The zero offset control compensates for sound transmission delays associated with the transducer, cable and couplant. This is a subtracted time measurement to compensate for the difference between the time data described below.

1. **Electric zero**: Point in time when the pulser fires the initial pulse to the transducer.
2. **Acoustic zero**: Point in time when the sound wave enters the test object.

Range Control

The range control enables the technician to set the visible A-scan screen range. Generally, the range should be set so the echo from the thickest material will be displayed on the screen. Successive presses of the range key toggle through preset range values, or the slewing keys can be held down to finely adjust the range setting, as shown in Figure 3.14.

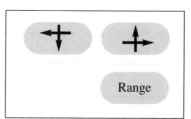

Figure 3.14: Press range then slewing keys to adjust range setting.

Range

Velocity Control

The velocity control adjusts the instrument settings to match the speed of sound in the test object. Velocity variables related to material density and elasticity, material temperature and mode, i.e., longitudinal wave versus shear wave, affect the velocity of sound within a given material. This control allows the technician to adjust the ultrasonic instrument based on the chosen mode of transmission, as well as the true velocity of that mode within the test object. This control is actuated much the same as the others, as shown in Figure 3.15.

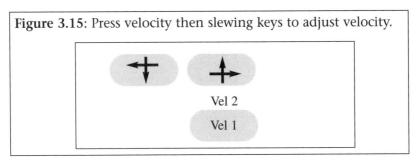

Figure 3.15: Press velocity then slewing keys to adjust velocity.

Vel 2

Vel 1

The gain controls the amplifier circuit to boost incoming signals from the material. There are several other controls provided in most ultrasonic instruments that work to modify the outbound pulses of energy or the display. These are referred to as *pulser settings*, and are as follows.

Rectification Control

This control adjusts the display signal on the screen. It adjusts the waveform display rectification between four selections: full wave rectify, half wave (+) rectify, half wave (–) rectify and radio frequency waveform (unrectified). Figure 3.16 provides examples of these four.

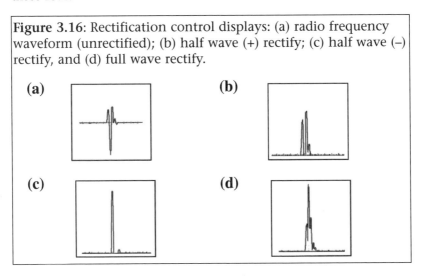

Figure 3.16: Rectification control displays: (a) radio frequency waveform (unrectified); (b) half wave (+) rectify; (c) half wave (–) rectify, and (d) full wave rectify.

(a)

(b)

(c)

(d)

Pulser Energy Control

The pulse of energy transmitted into the test object begins as an electrical impulse of low (100 V), medium (200 V) or high (400 V) voltage. The low voltage pulse produces better resolution, while the higher voltages produce greater penetrating power.

Damping Control

This control allows the technician to optimize waveform shape for high resolution measurements and for a particular transducer selection. The pulse duration is shortened or lengthened by its use. Typically, there are three setting options: 50 Ω for better near surface resolution, 150 Ω as a medium setting and 400 Ω for improved penetration.

Frequency Control

The frequency control allows for selection of a frequency setting that produces the desired screen presentation for the particular transducer chosen for the test application. Available frequencies are expressed in megahertz, and typically include 1, 2.25, 5, 10 and sometimes 15 MHz.

Other Features

Other controls might be included on an instrument, depending on the purchaser's desire for additional features. Such additional features may include some the following.

Distance Amplitude Correction

Distance amplitude correction (DAC), at times referred to as *time corrected gain* (TCG) or *time varied gain* depending on the manufacturer, is used to compensate for a drop in amplitude of signals reflected from discontinuities deep within the test object due to attenuation.

Gated Alarm

Gated alarm units enable automatic alarms when discontinuities are detected. This is accomplished by setting up specific, gated or zoned areas within the test object. Signals appearing within these gates may be monitored automatically to operate visual or audible alarms. These signals may also be passed to recorders and external control devices. Gated alarm units usually have three controls.

1. **Gate start or delay**: The gate start or delay control is used for adjustment of the location of the leading edge of the gate on the display screen.
2. **Gate length or width**: The gate length or width control is used for adjustment of the length of the gate or the location of the gate trailing edge.

3. **Gate alarm level or sensitivity**: The alarm level or gate level control is used for adjustment of the gate vertical threshold to turn on signal lights or to activate an alarm relay.

CALIBRATION

The first step in any ultrasonic test is to calibrate the instrument system to ensure proper performance. A predictable and reproducible response to known reflectors of different sizes and depths within the calibration standard must be demonstrated before any actual application to the test object can begin.

The calibration process amounts to an adjustment of the test system to the characteristic velocity and attenuation factor of material to be tested. Ideally, the calibration standard should be made of the same material as the test object, and should have been processed (including heat treating) identically to the test object. Further, the calibration standard, sometimes called a *calibration block*, should be adjusted to conform to the same temperature as that expected during the actual test.

Essentially, the calibration process is all about adjusting the ultrasonic test system so that it is capable of displaying signals from reflectors of known distance and size from the calibration standard. A properly calibrated test system will display linearity. That is, a reflector at a depth of 2.5 cm (1 in.) will cause a signal on the instrument display that can be easily read as being 2.5 cm (1 in.) deep.

The response of the instrument must be proportional to the size reflector, such that the technician will be readily able to see the difference between a signal from a reflector of 0.25 cm (0.1 in.) diameter versus one that is 0.3 cm (0.125 in.) in diameter. These and other details of calibration procedures are addressed in Chapter 7.

Basic Instrument Standardizing

A term less often used, but inherently more correct than calibrating, is *standardizing*. Standardizing the testing system is the adjustment of the equipment controls so that the technician can be sure that the instrument will detect the discontinuities that the test is expected to find. Standardizing the test system consists of setting up the instrument system exactly as it is to be used in the test, and adjusting the controls to give an adequate response to discontinuities of known size and depth in reference standards. The size and depth of the discontinuities are typically defined in a test specification.

Calibration Blocks

In ultrasonic testing, all discontinuity indications are compared to indications received from a reference standard. The reference standard may be any one of many reference blocks or sets of blocks specified for a given test.

Ultrasonic standard reference blocks, often called *calibration blocks*, are used in ultrasonic testing to standardize the ultrasonic equipment and to evaluate the discontinuity indication received from the test object. Standardizing does two things: it verifies that the instrument/transducer combination is performing with a proportional response; and it establishes a sensitivity or gain setting at which all discontinuities of a specified size or larger will be detected. Testing of discontinuities within the test object is accomplished by comparing their indications with the indication received from an artificial discontinuity of known size and at the same depth in a standard reference block of the same material.

Standard test blocks are made from carefully selected test stock that meets predetermined standards of sound attenuation, grain size and heat treatment. Discontinuities are represented by carefully drilled flat bottomed holes. Calibration blocks are made and tested with painstaking care so that the only discontinuity present is the one that was added intentionally. The most familiar sets of reference blocks are the Alcoa Series A area amplitude blocks.

Area amplitude blocks provide a means of checking the linearity of the output of the test system; that is, they confirm that the amplitude (height) of the indication on the display screen increases in proportion to the increase in size of the discontinuity. Similar area amplitude reference blocks are made from 5 cm (2 in.) diameter round stock.

Area Amplitude Blocks

The Alcoa Series A set consists of eight blocks, each 3-3/4 in. long and 1-15/16 in. square. A 3/4 in. deep flat bottomed hole is drilled in the bottom center of each block. The hole diameters are 1/64 in. in the number one block through 8/64 in. in the number eight block, as shown in Figure 3.17. As implied, the block numbers refer to the flat bottomed hole diameter (in fractions). For example, a number three block has a 3/64 in. diameter flat bottomed hole.

Area amplitude blocks provide a means of checking the proportional response of the test system; that is, they confirm that the amplitude (height) of the indication on the display screen increases in proportion to the increase in size of the discontinuity. Similar area amplitude reference blocks are made from 1-15/16 in. diameter round stock.

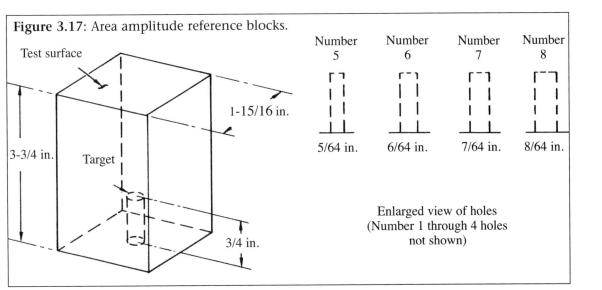

Figure 3.17: Area amplitude reference blocks.

Test surface

1-15/16 in.

3-3/4 in.

Target

3/4 in.

Number 5   Number 6   Number 7   Number 8

5/64 in.   6/64 in.   7/64 in.   8/64 in.

Enlarged view of holes
(Number 1 through 4 holes
not shown)

Distance Amplitude Blocks Set

The set of Alcoa Series B blocks consists of nineteen 1-15/16 in. diameter cylindrical blocks, all with 3/4 in. deep flat bottomed holes of the same diameter drilled in the center at one end. These blocks are of different lengths to provide metal distances of 1/16 to 5 3/4 in. from the test surface to the flat bottomed hole. Sets with 3/64, 5/64 or 8/64 in. diameter holes are available. The metal distances in each set are: 1/16 in.; 7/64 in. through 1 in. in 1/8 in. increments; and 1-1/4 in. through 5-3/4 in. in 1/2 in. increments. A set of these blocks is shown in Figure 3.18.

Distance amplitude blocks serve as a reference by which the size of discontinuities at varying depths within the test material may be evaluated. They also serve as a reference for setting or standardizing the sensitivity or gain of the test system so that the system will display readable indications on the display screen for all discontinuities of a given size and over, but will not flood the screen with indications of smaller discontinuities that are of no interest.

On instruments so equipped, distance amplitude blocks are used to set the sensitivity time control or distance amplitude correction so that a discontinuity of a given size will produce an indication of the same amplitude on the display screen, regardless of its distance from the front surface.

It is important that the test block material be the same or similar to that of the test object. Alloy content, heat treatment, degree of hot or cold working from forging, rolling, etc. all affect the acoustical properties of the material. If test blocks of identical material are not available, they must be similar in sound attenuation, velocity and impedance.

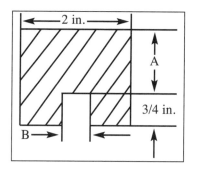

Figure 3.18: Distance amplitude reference blocks.

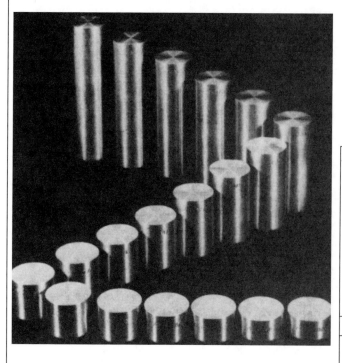

Dimension A	
1/16	1-3/4
1/8	2-1/4
1/4	2-3/4
3/8	3-1/4
1/2	3-3/4
5/8	4-1/4
3/4	4-3/4
7/8	5-1/4
1	5-1/4
1-1/4	

Dimension B
3/64
5/64
8/64

ASTM Calibration Blocks

Figure 3.19 shows an ASTM calibration block set. ASTM blocks can be combined into various sets of area amplitude and distance amplitude blocks. The ASTM basic set consists of ten 1-15/16 in. diameter blocks, each with a 5/64 in. deep flat bottom hole drilled in the center of the bottom surface. One block has a 3/64 in. diameter hole at a 3 in. metal distance. Seven blocks have 5/64 in. diameter holes at metal distances of 0.125, 0.25, 0.5, 0.75, 1.5, 3 and 6 in. The remaining blocks have 8/64 in. diameter holes at 3 in. and 6 in. metal distances. The three blocks with a 3 in. metal distance and hole diameters of 3/64, 5/64 and 8/64 in. form an area amplitude set, and the set with the 5/64 in. diameter holes provides a distance amplitude set.

In addition to the basic set, ASTM lists five more area amplitude standard reference blocks and 80 more distance amplitude blocks. Each ASTM block is identified by a code number, using the same system as that used for the Alcoa Series B set. The dimensions of all ASTM blocks are given in *ASTM Standard E-127*, which also presents the recommended steps for fabricating and checking aluminum alloy standard reference blocks. The recommended steps for fabricating and control of steel standard reference blocks

Figure 3.19: ASTM calibration block set.

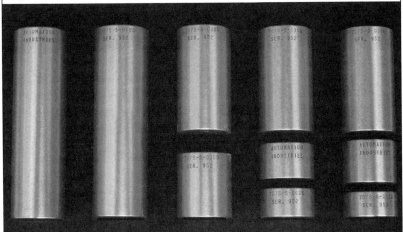

Figure 3.19: ASTM calibration block set.

are found in *ASTM Standard E-428*. Figure 3.20 provides an example of the construction of the ASTM calibration blocks.

It is important that the reference block material be the same or similar to that of the test object. Alloy content, heat treatment, degree of hot or cold working from forging and rolling all affect the acoustical properties of the material. If reference blocks of identical material are not available, they must be similar in sound attenuation, velocity and impedance.

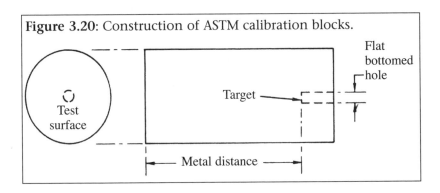

Figure 3.20: Construction of ASTM calibration blocks.

Special Blocks

The International Institute of Welding (IIW) reference block and the miniature angle beam field calibration block, shown in Figure 3.21, are examples of other reference standards in common use.

These standards are adequate for many test situations, provided the acoustic properties are matched or nearly matched between the test object and the test block. In most cases, responses from discontinuities in the test object are likely to differ from the indications received from the test block hole. For this reason, a sample test object is sectioned, subjected to metallurgical analysis and studied to determine the nature of the material and its probable discontinuities.

In some cases, artificial discontinuities in the form of holes or notches are introduced into the sample to serve as a basis for comparison with discontinuities found in other test objects. From these studies, an acceptance level is determined that establishes the number and magnitude of discontinuities allowed in the test object. In all cases, the true nature of the test material is determined by careful study of the sample test object; and a sensible testing program is established by an intelligent application of basic theory.

For irregularly shaped test objects, it is often necessary to make one of the test objects into a reference standard by adding artificial discontinuities in the form of flat bottomed holes, saw cuts, notches, etc. In some cases, these artificial discontinuities can be placed so that they will be removed by subsequent machining of the test object. In other cases, a special individual standardizing technique is developed by carefully studying a test object ultrasonically, and then verifying the detection of discontinuities in the test object by destructive investigation. The results of the study then become the basis for the testing standard.

Figure 3.21: Special reference blocks.

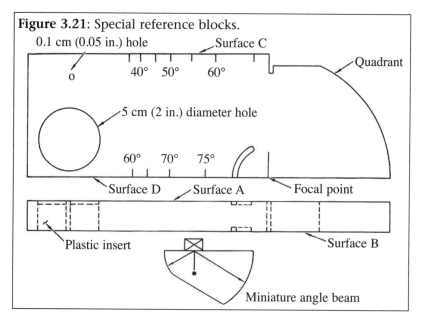

Digital Thickness Instrumentation

Ultrasonic instrumentation manufacturers initiated their move away from vacuum tube analog instruments and toward digital technology in the late 1960s. Some of the earliest representations of the trend were built to satisfy a need to produce small instruments that could be used to acquire thickness readings from plate, as well as pressured pipe and vessel walls.

The early units represented the results of the test by use of needle pointers that would swing to a point on a dial to indicate wall thickness. Next came the digital display units that used small vacuum tubes capable of displaying numbers from zero through nine. With three or four of these tubes arranged horizontally, a technician could directly read the results of each thickness test in the numbers illuminated with the tubes. The current generation of the digital meters use liquid crystal displays to provide the information.

Modern ultrasonic thickness gages may be used to measure wall thickness of metals, glass, ceramics and rigid plastics. They use the pulse echo principle of ultrasonic application, where short pulses of energy are transmitted from a high frequency transducer into the test object. The emitted pulses travel through the material to its inside surface and reflect back to the transducer. The elapsed travel time for the completion of the round trip is measured and converted to an accurate digital thickness measurement.

Today's digital thickness meters are small and light weight, and are capable of producing very accurate results. Most provide data logging capacity that allows for easy information gathering and transfer to computer based data analysis programs.

Figure 3.22 shows a digital thickness meter that is small, and yet powerful in its ability to resolve and accurately display wall thickness readings of various materials. It displays only the thickness value, but does not provide an A-scan display.

Figure 3.22: Thickness meter with liquid crystal display screen.

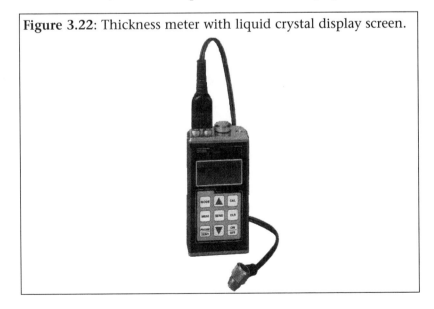

In the mid 1980s, several manufacturers developed a new generation of the digital meters that use liquid crystal displays to provide waveform information on A-scan displays, in addition to the digital readout of the thickness value. The A-scan displays enable the technician to view the waveform and decide whether the digital thickness value presented results from an internal reflector or the actual inside wall of the test object. Such a unit is shown in Figure 3.23.

Figure 3.23: Thickness meter with A-scan and digital display.

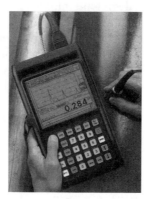

Chapter 4

Transducer Operation and Theory

INTRODUCTION

In ultrasonic testing, the essential sensor of the system is the transducer. As seen in Figure 4.1, the transducer is a combination of several elements. It performs many functions, all centering around the piezoelectric element and the work it performs.

Figure 4.1: Transducer components.

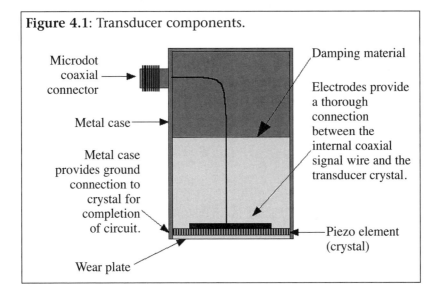

Microdot coaxial connector

Metal case

Metal case provides ground connection to crystal for completion of circuit.

Wear plate

Damping material

Electrodes provide a thorough connection between the internal coaxial signal wire and the transducer crystal.

Piezo element (crystal)

Piezoelectric Effect

Piezoelectricity is a property of certain crystalline materials including natural crystals of quartz, rochelle salt and tourmaline, plus manufactured ceramics such as barium titanate and lead zirconate titanates.

The prefix *piezo* is derived from a Greek word meaning *to press*. When mechanical pressure is applied to one of these materials, the crystalline structure produces a voltage proportional to the pressure. Conversely, when an electric field is applied, the structure changes shape producing dimensional changes in the material.

To produce an ultrasonic beam in a test object, a component of an ultrasonic instrument, called a *pulser*, applies high frequency electrical pulses through a coaxial cable to a piezoelectric crystal contained inside of the transducer.

Transducer Materials

Early developers of ultrasonic transducers found that naturally occurring quartz crystal, when sliced into a very thin wafer and shaped into a coin-like disk, worked nicely to produce the conversion bridge required to transmit and receive energy to and from the materials they were testing. The three most common piezoelectric materials used in ultrasonic transducers from the 1930s through the early 1980s were quartz, polarized ceramic, barium titanate and lithium sulfate. Barium titanate was regarded as the best material to use as a transmitting crystal, while lithium sulfate was widely thought to be the best material for receiving ultrasonic vibrations. Today, the most common crystalline components of the ceramic transducer elements are barium titanate, lead metaniobate and lead zirconate titanate.

Since the early 1980s, ultrasonic crystal elements have changed in an important way. The ability to manufacture designer crystals by use of ceramic technology has improved on the natural crystals found in nature. Now, barium titanate, lead zirconate, lead titanate and many others are available in precision molded ceramic wafers that demonstrate improved performance compared to the older natural crystals.

The composition, shape and dimensions of a piezoelectric ceramic element can now be tailored to meet the requirements of a specific purpose. Ceramics manufactured from formulations of lead zirconate and lead titanate (known as *PZT materials*) exhibit greater sensitivity and higher operating temperatures, relative to ceramics of other compositions, and currently are the most widely used piezoelectric elements. The phrase *polarized ceramic* is commonly used to describe these newer ultrasonic elements.

Frequency

The frequency of a transducer is a determining factor in its use. For example, a technician making thickness determinations on thin wall 0.15 cm (0.06 in.) tubing would choose a 10 MHz transducer to gain its ability to resolve signals returning from very short distances. A technician performing shear wave inspection would probably prefer to use a 2.25 MHz frequency transducer, which would provide a combination of good sensitivity and good penetrating ability because its wavelength is longer than that produced by a higher frequency.

A technician may choose a given frequency transducer based on the sensitivity that a project specification requires. (Sensitivity is related to wavelength: the higher the frequency, the shorter the wavelength, which produces better sensitivity.) So a higher frequency is required if the technician is concerned with obtaining higher levels of sensitivity.

Most ultrasonic testing is performed using frequencies between 0.2 and 25 MHz, with contact testing generally limited to 10 MHz and below because crystals ground for use above 10 MHz are too thin and fragile for practical contact testing. Transducer frequency and crystal thickness are integrally related: the thinner the crystal, the higher the frequency; the thicker the crystal, the lower the frequency. Other considerations for selection of a given transducer for a specific job include the following.

1. The higher the frequency of a transducer, the straighter (less beam spread) the sound beam and the greater the sensitivity and resolution, but the attenuation is also greater and the penetration is poor.
2. The lower the frequency of a transducer, the deeper the penetration and the less the attenuation, but the greater the beam spread, the less the sensitivity and resolution.
3. At any given frequency, the larger the transducer, the straighter the sound beam, but the less sensitivity.
4. When testing cast metallic materials that have coarse grain structures, lower frequencies of no more than 1 to 2.25 MHz are required in order to penetrate to the opposite surface. Even lower frequencies (down to 200 kHz) are required for ultrasonic tests of wood and concrete.

NEAR FIELD AND FAR FIELD

In ultrasonic testing, the sonic beam is generally considered to be a straight sided projection of the face of the transducer. In reality, the beam is not very consistent. By setting up a transducer in an immersion tank, the beam intensity can be measured in the water at various distances from the transducer face. Using this technique, two distinct zones are always present within the sonic beam. These zones are known as the *near field*, or *Fresnel zone*, and the *far field*, or *Fraunhofer zone*. The near field and far field are illustrated in Figure 4.2.

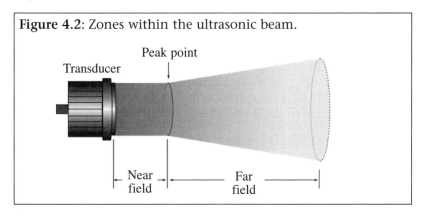

Figure 4.2: Zones within the ultrasonic beam.

Peak point

Transducer

Near field

Far field

Near Field

In the zone closest to the transducer, the measurement of the ultrasonic intensities reveals an irregular pattern of localized high and low intensities. This irregular pattern results from the interference between sound waves that are emitted from the face of the transducer. The transducer may be considered to be a mosaic of crystals, each vibrating at the same frequency but slightly out of phase with each other. Near the face of the crystal, the composite sound beam propagates chiefly as a plane front wave. However, the spherical front waves, which emanate from the periphery of the crystal face, produce side lobe waves that interfere with the plane front waves. This causes patterns of acoustical maximums and minimums where they cross, as shown in Figure 4.3.

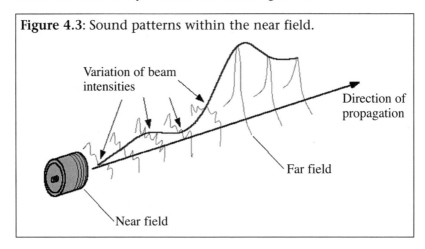

Figure 4.3: Sound patterns within the near field.

The effect of these acoustical patterns in the near zone varies during an ultrasonic test. However, if the technician has proper knowledge of the near field, the correct reference block can be scanned and correlated with the indications from the test.

The length of the near field is dependent on the diameter of the transducer and the wavelength of the ultrasonic beam, and may be computed from Eq. 4.1.

Eq. 4.1 $L = \dfrac{D^2}{4\lambda}$

where L is the length of the near field, D is the diameter of the transducer and λ is the wavelength of the ultrasonic energy.

Since the wavelength of ultrasonic energy in a particular material is inversely proportional to the frequency, the length of the near field in a particular material can be shortened by lowering the frequency.

Far Field

In the zone furthest from the transducer, the only effect of consequence is the spreading of the ultrasonic beam and the natural attenuation effect of the material. As shown in Figure 4.2, the highest sound intensity occurs at the end of the near field/beginning of the far field. From that point on, the beam intensity is reduced by the attenuation characteristics of the material in which it is traveling and by beam spread.

Beam Spread

Fraunhofer diffraction causes the beam to spread starting at the end of the near field. At this distance, the beam originates at the center of the radiating face of the transducer and spreads outward, as shown in Figure 4.4.

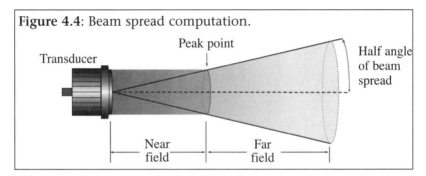

Figure 4.4: Beam spread computation.

The degree of spread may be computed using Eq. 4.2.

Eq. 4.2 $\sin \theta = 1.22 \dfrac{\lambda}{D}$

where θ is the half angle of spread, λ is the wavelength of the ultrasonic energy and D is the diameter of the transducer.

At any frequency, the larger the crystal, the straighter the beam; the smaller the crystal, the greater the beam spread. Also, there is less beam spread for the same diameter of crystal at higher frequencies than at lower frequencies. The diameter of the transducer is often limited by the size of the available contact surface. Transducers as small as 0.32 cm (0.125 in.) diameter have been used. For shallow depth testing, 1 cm (0.38 in.) and 1.3 cm (0.5 in.) diameter transducers are used at the higher frequencies, such as 5 to 25 MHz. A large diameter transducer is usually selected for testing through greater depths of material.

Table 4.1 shows that as frequency is increased, and as transducer diameter is increased, beam spread is decreased. Conversely, as frequency is decreased, and as transducer diameter is decreased, beam spread increases. The ultrasonic technician must choose a transducer carefully to fit the job at hand. The proper combination of frequency and diameter has a strong influence on the success of the test.

Table 4.1: Beam spread in steel.		Transducer diameter (inch)			
Frequency (megahertz)	λ (inch)	0.375	0.5	1.95	2.54
1	0.2287	48° 10'	34°	21° 52'	16° 13'
2.25	0.102	19° 23'	14° 25'	9° 33'	7° 9'
5	0.0457	8° 34'	6° 25'	4° 16'	3° 12'

Side Lobe Radiation

In addition to the main beam of ultrasonic energy, the side lobe beams of ultrasonic energy are sometimes generated by the piezoelectric element (crystal). Side lobe beams are produced as a function of transducer diameter and frequency. These waves may travel parallel to the test surface. Figure 4.5 illustrates this phenomenon. If possible, the technician selects transducers that minimize side lobes, and the primary beam is the only one of consequence. Side lobe beams must be considered when the geometry of the test object is such that they are reflected back to the transducer, creating spurious effects such as the generation of reflections from the nearby top corner edges of a test object.

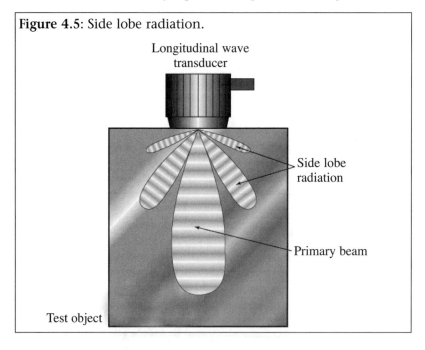

Figure 4.5: Side lobe radiation.

Types of Transducers

Transducers are made in a limitless number of sizes and shapes, from extremely small (0.02 cm [0.008 in.] diameter) to 15 cm (6 in.) wide paintbrush transducers. The many shapes are the result of much experience and the requirement for many special applications. Size of a transducer is a contributing factor to its performance. For instance, the larger the transducer, the straighter the sound beam (less beam spread) for a given frequency. The narrower beams of the small, high frequency transducers have greater ability for detecting very small discontinuities. The larger transducers transmit more sound energy into the test object, so they are used to gain deep penetration. The large, single crystal transducers are generally limited to lower frequencies because the very thin, high frequency transducers are susceptible to breaking and chipping.

Paintbrush Transducers

Wide paintbrush transducers are made up of a mosaic pattern of smaller crystals carefully matched so that the intensity of the beam pattern varies very little over the entire length of the transducer. This is necessary to maintain uniform sensitivity. Paintbrush transducers provide a long, narrow, rectangular beam (in cross-section) for scanning large surfaces. Their purpose is to quickly discover discontinuities in the test object. Smaller, more sensitive transducers are then used to define the size, shape, orientation and exact location of the discontinuities. Figure 4.6 shows a typical paintbrush transducer.

Figure 4.6: Paintbrush transducer.

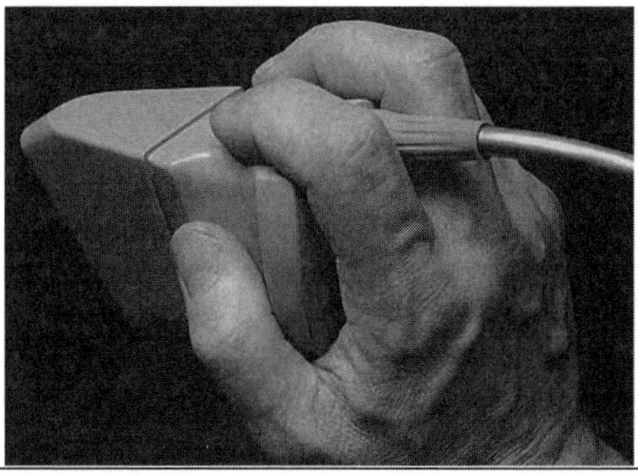

Dual Transducers

Dual transducers differ from single transducers in that two piezoelectric elements are used. Whereas the single transducer may be a transmitter only, a receiver only or both transmitter and receiver, the dual transducer is essentially two single transducers mounted in the same holder for pitch and catch testing. In the dual transducer, one transducer is the transmitter and the other is the receiver. They may be mounted side by side for longitudinal wave testing, and stacked or paired side by side for shear wave testing. In all cases, the crystals are separated by a sound barrier to block cross talk interference. Figure 4.7 shows both types of dual transducers.

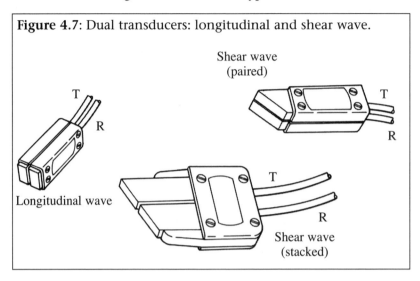

Figure 4.7: Dual transducers: longitudinal and shear wave.

Shear Wave Transducers

Transducers are also classified as either longitudinal wave transducers or shear wave transducers. The term longitudinal means that the sound energy from the transducer is transmitted into the test object in a direction perpendicular to the test surface. An often substituted name for longitudinal wave is *straight beam*.

Shear wave transducers direct the sound beam into the test surface at an angle that is not perpendicular. An often substituted name for shear wave is *angle beam*. Shear wave transducers are used to locate discontinuities oriented at angles to the surface and to determine the size of discontinuities oriented at angles between 90° and 180° to the surface.

Angled plastic (usually acrylic polymer) shoes are mechanically attached to longitudinal wave transducers to propagate shear, surface or plate waves into the test object by mode conversion. In contact testing, angle beam transducers use a wedge, usually made of plastic, between the transducer face and the surface of the test object to direct the sound energy into the test surface at the desired angle. In immersion testing, control of the sound beam into the test object at the desired angle is accomplished by means of an adjustable angle transducer holder. Both straight and angled transducers are shown in Figure 4.8.

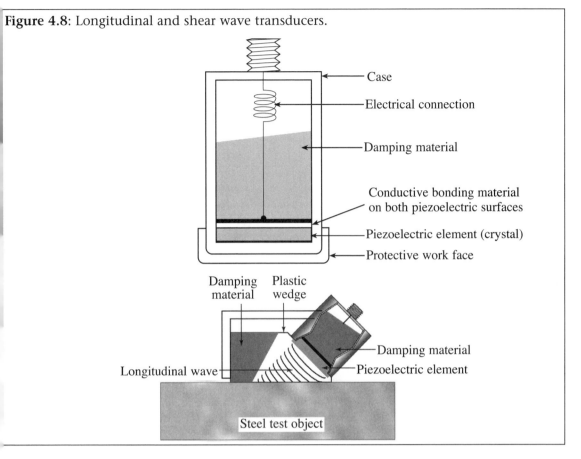

Figure 4.8: Longitudinal and shear wave transducers.

Case

Electrical connection

Damping material

Conductive bonding material
on both piezoelectric surfaces

Piezoelectric element (crystal)

Protective work face

Damping material   Plastic wedge

Damping material

Longitudinal wave   Piezoelectric element

Steel test object

Faced Unit or Contour Focused Transducers

In addition to wedges, other frontal members are added to the transducer for various reasons. On contact transducers, wear plates are often added to protect the front electrode and to protect the fragile crystal from wear, breakage or the harmful effects of foreign substances or liquids. (Notice the protective wear face of the longitudinal transducer in Figure 4.8.)

Frontal units shaped to direct the sound energy perpendicular to the surface at all points on curved surfaces are known as *contour correction lenses*. These cylindrical lenses sharpen the front surface indication by evening out the sound travel distance between the transducer and the test surface. A comparison of flat and contoured transducers is shown in Figure 4.9.

Other acoustic lenses focus the sound beam from the transducer. Focused transducers concentrate the sound energy into a narrow, sharp pointed beam of increased intensity, which is capable of detecting very small discontinuities in a relatively small area. Focusing the sound beam moves its point of maximum intensity toward the transducer, but shortens its usable range. The test object has the effect of a second lens because the beam is refracted, as shown in Figure 4.10, when the beam enters the test surface.

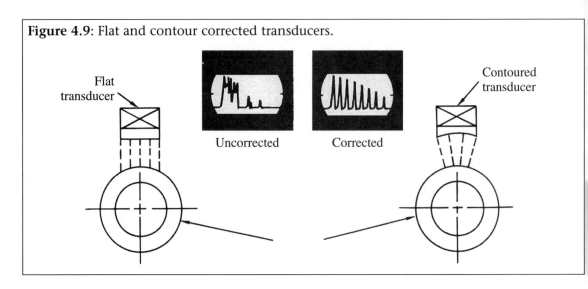

Figure 4.9: Flat and contour corrected transducers.

Flat transducer

Uncorrected   Corrected

Contoured transducer

The increased intensity produces increased sensitivity. Moving the point of maximum intensity closer to the transducer (which is also closer to the test surface) improves the near surface resolution. The disturbing effects of rough surface and metal noise are also reduced by concentrating the sound energy into a smaller beam. This is because a smaller area is being looked at. In a smaller area, the true discontinuity indications are relatively large compared to the combined noise of other nonrelevant indications. The useful thickness range of focused transducers is about 0.03 to 5 cm (0.01 to 2 in.).

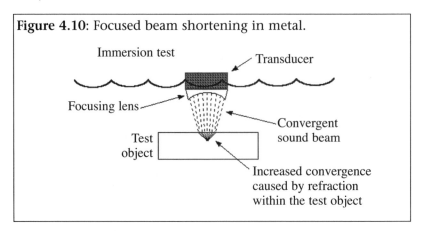

Figure 4.10: Focused beam shortening in metal.

Immersion test   Transducer

Focusing lens

Test object

Convergent sound beam

Increased convergence caused by refraction within the test object

Electronically Focused Transducers

Special transducers, known as *linear arrays* or *phased arrays*, can be focused using electronic phase control. A typical linear array is shown in Figure 4.11. The linear array is a collection of very small transducers, with each transducer able to act as a transmitter or receiver. Transducer width may be as small as 0.05 cm (0.02 in.), and an array may consist of several hundred small transducers. By

Figure 4.11: Linear array may be built to contain almost any number of transducers, and may be built to any shape required to perform a specific test.

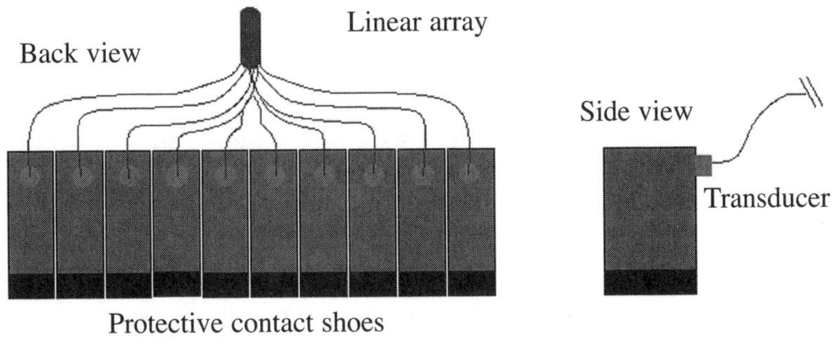

Back view
Linear array

Side view

Transducer

Protective contact shoes

selectively pulsing each transducer or group of transducers in a given order, the ultrasonic beam may be focused in depth, or may cause the focused beam to sweep across the test object without moving the array.

Contact Transducers

Contact transducers are made for both straight beam and angle beam testing. Figure 4.12 illustrates the construction of a longitudinal wave contact transducer, and also pictures another longitudinal wave transducer that is designed to screw into a plastic wedge to be used for shear wave testing.

Figure 4.12: Contact transducer construction.

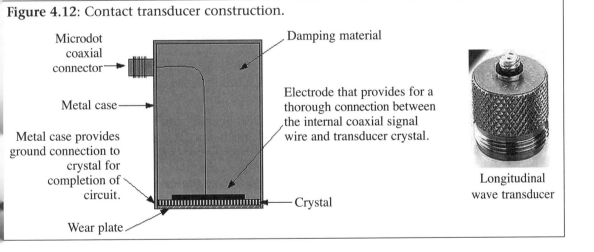

Microdot coaxial connector

Damping material

Metal case

Electrode that provides for a thorough connection between the internal coaxial signal wire and transducer crystal.

Metal case provides ground connection to crystal for completion of circuit.

Crystal

Wear plate

Longitudinal wave transducer

Beam Intensity Characteristics

The strongest intensity of the sound beam is along its central axis, with a gradual reduction in amplitude away from the axis. In the near field, the measurement of the sonic intensities reveals an irregular pattern of localized high and low intensities. This irregular pattern results from the interference between sound waves that are emitted from the face of the transducer. The effect that the presence of these acoustical patterns in the near field will have on the ultrasonic test varies, but if the technician has accurate knowledge of the length of the near field, the proper test block can be scanned and correlated to those indications that originate from within the test object.

In the zone furthest from the transducer (the far field or Fraunhofer zone), the only effect of consequence is the spreading of the ultrasonic beam and the natural attenuation effect of the material.

SENSITIVITY, RESOLUTION AND DAMPING

The capabilities of a transducer, and for that matter the testing system, are for the most part described by two terms: sensitivity and resolution.

Sensitivity

The sensitivity of a transducer is its ability to detect echoes from small discontinuities. Transducer sensitivity is measured by the amplitude of its response from an artificial discontinuity in a standard reference block. Precise transducer sensitivity is unique to a specific transducer. Even transducers of the same size, frequency and material by the same manufacturer do not always produce identical indications on a given display screen. A transducer's sensitivity is rated by its ability to detect a given size flat bottomed hole at a specific depth in a standard reference block.

Resolution

The resolution or resolving power of a transducer refers to its ability to separate the echoes from two reflectors close together in time; for example, the front surface echo and an echo from a small discontinuity just beneath the surface. The time required for the transducer to stop ringing or vibrating after having been supplied with a long voltage pulse is a measure of its near surface resolving power. Long tails or wave trains of sound energy from a ringing transducer cause a wide, high amplitude echo from all reflectors in the sound path, including the entry surface.

As illustrated in Figure 4.13a, a small discontinuity just beneath the surface is easily masked by the ringing signal of the initial pulse. Figure 4.13 shows that even reflectors at a greater distance are not displayed distinctly due to the same issue of too long a pulse length applied to the transducer. Figure 4.14 displays examples of poor versus good resolution in the far field.

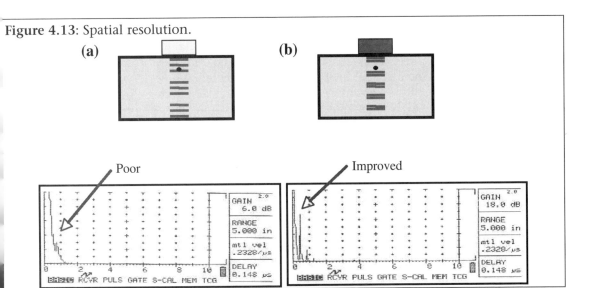

Figure 4.13: Spatial resolution.

(a)

(b)

Poor

Improved

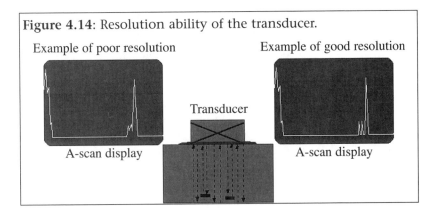

Figure 4.14: Resolution ability of the transducer.

Example of poor resolution

Example of good resolution

A-scan display

Transducer

A-scan display

Spatial Resolution

Spatial resolution relates to the ability of a transducer to differentiate between two or more reflectors that are closely spaced in a lateral plane perpendicular to the axis of sound beam propagation, as shown in Figure 4.15. Spatial resolution is a function of the transducer's characteristic near field and beam spread.

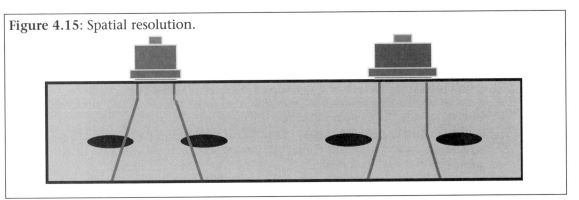

Figure 4.15: Spatial resolution.

Damping

Damping refers to the time required for the crystal to quit vibrating after excitation. The resolution of the transducer is directly related to the damping time. The lesser the damping time, the better the ability of the transducer to resolve two signals arriving close together at a given time, or to resolve signals from near the contact test surface. Figure 4.16 illustrates a so-called *dead zone* that takes up one tenth of the total screen range. Transducer damping and instrument setting are factors shown here.

Figure 4.16: Transducer damping.

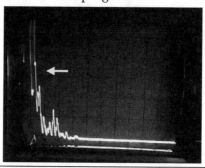

Other Types of Transducers

Historically, ultrasonic transducers have required a direct link to the test object. The transducer had to be in intimate contact with the test object and be coupled by a liquid. In the case of direct contact techniques involving the scanning of large, very rough or high temperature surfaces, this coupling results in transducers being damaged by mechanical wear or by temperatures above 100 °C (212 °F). Several noncontacting transducers have been developed. It must be noted that the noncontacting feature comes with certain constraints. For example, there is a drastic decrease in signal strength and signal-to-noise ratios in comparison to typical piezoelectric transducers.

Electromagnetic Acoustic Transducers

The development of this noncontacting type of transducer has provided new and important opportunities for ultrasonic testing. EMAT is an acronym for electromagnetic acoustic transducer. Electromagnetic acoustic transducers can generate longitudinal, shear, plate and surface waves in metallic test objects.

Practical electromagnetic probes consist of a coil wound into a geometrical shape to create a specific mechanical disturbance pattern. The probe also contains a magnet to aid the consistent vertical orientation to the test surface. Since many coil and magnet configurations are possible, many variations of wave patterns have been generated. Figure 4.17 shows one configuration that generates a 0° shear wave useful for thickness gaging.

Figure 4.17: Zero degree electromagnetic acoustic transducer.

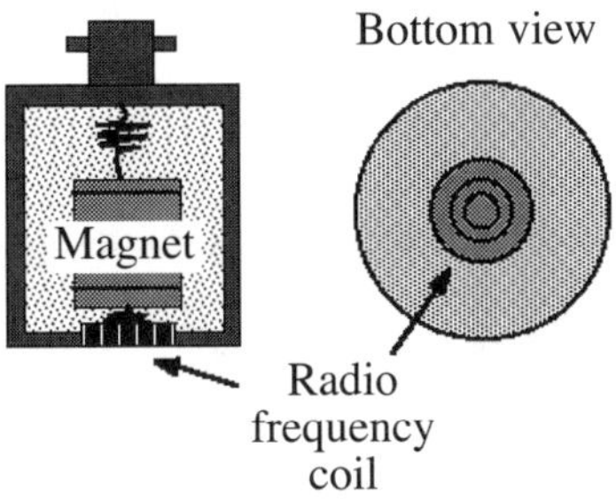

Operating frequencies can be as high as 20 MHz, limiting thickness testing applications to material having wall thickness greater than about 0.1 cm (0.04 in.). The coil diameter, wire size and magnet size depend on the application and the current available for driving the transducer. This type of transducer is used for thickness gaging in high speed automatic testing stations.

Electromagnetic acoustic transducers are useful at elevated temperatures for testing metals in the early stages of forming, even while the material is red hot. Although it usually requires the addition of cooling systems for the transducer assembly (coil and magnet), EMAT technology is proving itself successful as a standard testing application for improving the quality of the finishes products of the mills.

Electromagnetic acoustic transducers are also effective when high speed testing is needed, as in the case of pipeline tests and railroad wheels. Remote tests of pipelines have been performed from the inside using electromagnetic acoustic transducers and remotely controlled robots called *pigs*. The electromagnetic acoustic transducer's ability to launch Lamb or plate waves results in indications of corrosion where the thickness of the pipe has been modified, as it often is near circumferential welds.

Being electrically controlled devices, electromagnetic acoustic transducers lend themselves to phased array technology when modifications of the interrogating ultrasonic beams might improve testing. Where test objects must remain in a vacuum, as in electron beam welding, electromagnetic acoustic transducers perform well.

The principle disadvantage that has been discovered while using EMATs is that relatively low amounts of ultrasonic energy can be transmitted into the material due to the air interference. This relative inefficiency often yields lower signal-to-noise ratios than can be achieved with conventional probes. Every problem relative to use of EMATs has not been eliminated, but scientists are working toward improving several issues that will, once solved, broaden the applicability of this relatively new ultrasonic testing application.

Air Coupled Transducers

An immerging technology that brings promise to the broader application of ultrasonic testing is one that uses air (no liquid) as the coupling medium. All the restrictions that relate to the transmission of ultrasound through a low density material such as air have been managed to a degree that the technology can be applied as another ultrasonic testing tool. Relatively low frequency (under 200 kHz) transducers designed to acoustically match the impedance value of air are key elements to this new approach. The transducers are designed to yield relatively large mechanical displacements in air.

Due to the low acoustic velocity of air, relatively small wavelengths can be achieved but they are quickly attenuated when transmitted. Much of the science that has allowed this new technology to develop has centered around improved pulser and receiver circuits within the instruments, and transducers designed to transmit sound efficiently into air.

Thus far, most applications have been done to low impedance materials such as honeycomb composite structures using the through transmission mode. Figure 4.17 shows several of the low frequency (400 KHz down to 50 KHz) transducers.

Figure 4.18: Low frequency air coupled transducers.

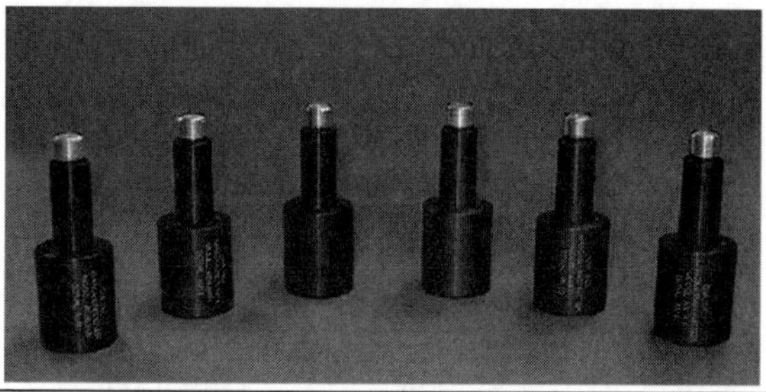

Laser Induced Ultrasound

Still another approach for introducing ultrasound into a test object without physical contact takes advantage of the energy stored in a short duration pulse from a high energy laser. A mechanical wave is generated by thermal expansion that takes place at the surface contacted by a laser beam. The expansion that takes place is oriented normal to the surface and therefore creates a longitudinal wave within the material.

Shorter pulses yield short duration mechanical disturbances and higher frequency ultrasonic waves. Regardless of the angle the laser beam impinges on the test object, the resulting sound beam travels within the test object in a direction that is normal to that surface. This makes it possible for laser induced ultrasound to be effective at finding laminar discontinuities, even in curved test objects. Noncontacting and remote systems have been successfully developed using optical interferometers as the receiving sensor. As with electromagnetic acoustic transducers and air coupled devices, the acoustic energy is very small, and these systems tend to exhibit poor signal-to-noise ratios.

Air coupled, laser coupled and EMAT technologies are still in their infancy compared to contact and immersion testing. The discussions and general examples that are used throughout this book relate to requirements for thorough coupling by use of denser materials, such as liquid.

More information on these transducers and the new techniques that have been made possible by their development is provided in Chapter 5.

COUPLANTS

Purpose and Principles

As noted in previous chapters, one of the practical problems in ultrasonic testing is the transmission of the ultrasonic energy from the source into the test object. If a transducer is placed in contact with the surface of a dry test object, very little energy is transmitted through the interface into the material because of the presence of air between the transducer and the test material. The air causes a great difference in acoustic impedance at the interface. This is called an *impedance mismatch*.

Typically, a couplant is used between the transducer face and the test surface to ensure efficient sound transmission from transducer to test surface. The couplant, as the name implies, couples the transducer ultrasonically to the surface of the test object by filling in the gaps between the irregularities of the test surface and the transducer face, thus excluding all air from between the transducer and the test surface.

Materials

The couplant can be any of a vast variety of liquids, semiliquids, pastes and even some solids that will satisfy the following requirements.

1. A couplant wets (fully contacts) both the surface of the test object and the face of the transducer and excludes all air from between them.
2. A couplant is easy to apply.
3. A couplant is homogeneous and free of air bubbles, or solid particles in the case of a nonsolid.
4. A couplant is harmless to the test object and transducer.
5. A couplant has a tendency to stay on the test surface, but it is easy to remove when the test is complete.

Contact Couplant Selection

In contact testing, the choice of couplant depends primarily on the test conditions, such as the condition of the test surface (rough or smooth), the temperature of the test surface and the position of the test surface (horizontal, slanted or vertical).

One part glycerin with two parts water and a wetting agent is often used on relatively smooth, horizontal surfaces. For slightly rough surfaces, light oils with an added wetting agent are used. Rough surfaces, hot surfaces and vertical surfaces require a heavier oil or grease as a couplant. In all cases, the couplant selected should meet the five criteria listed above.

Immersion Couplant Selection

In immersion testing, clean, deaerated tap water is used for a couplant. For technician comfort, the water temperature is usually maintained at 21 °C (70 °F) by automatic controls. Wetting agents are added to the water to ensure that the surface is thoroughly wet, thereby eliminating air bubbles.

Chapter 5

Basic Ultrasonic Testing Methods

INTRODUCTION

The type of test required for a particular component is usually given in a specification that tells the technician the type of discontinuities to look for, the type of test required to locate the discontinuities and the limits of acceptability. The specification typically provides other basic facts pertinent to the test. It is up to the technician to follow the specification. The sections that follow are intended to familiarize the technician with the basic steps that are required to conduct satisfactory ultrasonic tests.

Once the testing system is standardized, the actual testing can begin. With the exception of the gain controls, the test instrument controls are not to be adjusted during actual testing because adjusting the controls negates the standardization and requires restandardization of the instrument.

CONTACT TESTING

Methods of ultrasonic testing are accomplished with one of two basic techniques: contact testing or immersion testing. In contact testing, the transducer is placed in direct contact with the test object with a thin liquid film used as a couplant. On some contact units, plastic wedges, wear plates or flexible membranes are mounted over the face of the crystal. Transducer units are considered to be "in contact" whenever the sound beam is transmitted through a couplant other than water. The display from a contact unit usually shows the initial pulse and the front surface reflection as superimposed or very close together.

Contact testing is divided into four techniques that are determined by the sound beam wave mode: (1) transmitting longitudinal waves in the test object; (2) generating shear waves; (3) producing Rayleigh (or surface) waves; and (4) producing Lamb (or plate) waves. Transducers used in these techniques are held in direct contact with the material using a thin liquid film as a couplant. The couplant is high enough in viscosity to remain on the test surface during the test. For most contact testing, the couplant is relatively thin. Refer to Chapter 4 for more information on contact transducers and couplants.

Longitudinal Wave Technique

The longitudinal wave technique is accomplished by projecting a sound beam perpendicularly to the surface of the test object to obtain pulse echo reflections from the back surface or from discontinuities that lie between the two surfaces. This technique is also used in through transmission application using two transducers where the internal discontinuities interrupt the sound beam, causing a reduction in the received signal.

Pulse Echo Techniques

Pulse echo techniques may use either single or double crystal transducers. Figure 5.1 shows the single crystal, longitudinal wave transducer in use. The single crystal transducer acts as both transmitter and receiver, projecting a pulsed beam of longitudinal waves into the test object and receiving echoes reflected from the back surface and from any discontinuity lying in the beam path. The double crystal transducer is useful when the test material thickness is relatively thin (less that 0.5 in.), when the test surface is rough or when the test object shape is irregular and the back surface is not parallel with the front surface. One transducer transmits and the other receives, as shown in Figure 5.2. In this case, the receiver unit is receiving back surface and discontinuity echoes, even though the transmitter unit is not directly over the reflectors.

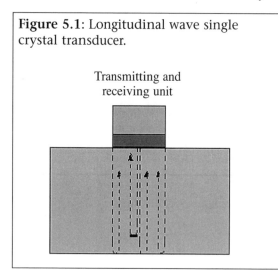

Figure 5.1: Longitudinal wave single crystal transducer.

Transmitting and receiving unit

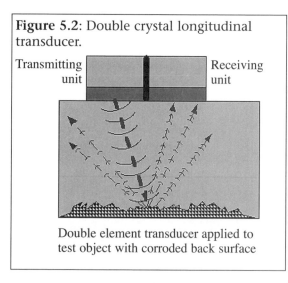

Figure 5.2: Double crystal longitudinal transducer.

Transmitting unit

Receiving unit

Double element transducer applied to test object with corroded back surface

Through Transmission Technique

With the through transmission technique, two transducers are used, one on each side of the test object, as shown in Figure 5.3. One unit acts as a transmitter, and the other as a receiver. The transmitter unit projects a sound beam into the material, the beam travels through the material to the opposite surface and the sound is picked up at the opposite surface by the receiving unit. Any discontinuities in the path of the sound beam cause a reduction in the amount of sound energy reaching the receiving unit. For best results in this technique, the transmitter unit selected is the best available generator of acoustic energy, and the receiver unit selected is the best available receiver of acoustic energy. A barium titanate transmitter used with a lithium sulfate receiver would have been common until the early 1980s, but many new piezoelectric ceramic crystal materials have been perfected since that time. These are discussed in Chapter 6.

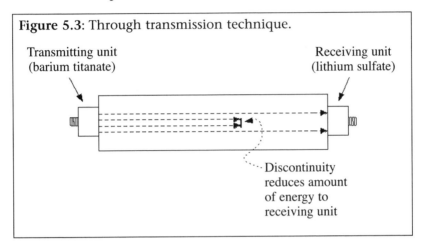

Figure 5.3: Through transmission technique.

Angle Beam Transmission Technique

The angle beam technique is used to transmit sound waves into the test object at a predetermined angle to the test surface. Depending on the angle selected, the wave modes produced in the test object may be refracted longitudinal and shear waves, shear waves only or surface wave (Rayleigh) mode. Of these options, it is the shear wave technique that is most often applied to ultrasonic testing, particularly as it applies to weld inspection. Figure 5.4 illustrates a shear wave application scanning plate and pipe material.

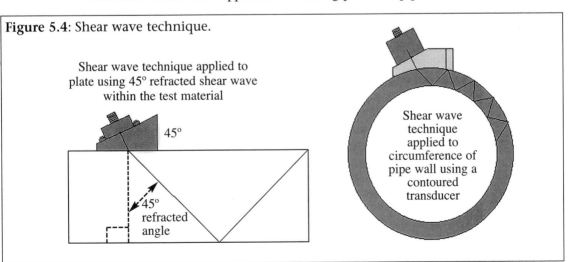

Figure 5.4: Shear wave technique.

Surface Wave Technique

Angle beam techniques are used for testing welds, pipe or tubing, sheet and plate material and for test objects of irregular shape where straight beam units are unable to contact all of the surface. Angle beam transducers are identified by case markings that show sound beam direction by an arrow and that indicate the angle of refraction in steel for shear waves.

Angles of incidence may cause the refracted wave within the test material to become a surface (or Rayleigh) wave. This wave mode travels only at or near (within three wavelengths) the surface of a solid material, and exhibits a completely different wave motion than that of longitudinal or shear waves. The creation of a surface wave using a plastic transducer wedge requires that the incident angle in the wedge is greater than the second critical angel. In the case of test objects prone to near surface discontinuities, especially where the test surface is fairly smooth, surface wave techniques offer excellent testing results. Figure 5.5 illustrates this technique. Note the particle motion that the wave causes within the test material compared to that of the longitudinal or shear waves.

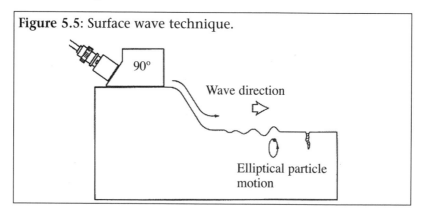

Figure 5.5: Surface wave technique.

90°

Wave direction

Elliptical particle motion

IMMERSION TESTING

In immersion testing, a waterproof transducer is used at some distance from the test object, and the ultrasonic beam is transmitted into the material through a water path or column. The water distance appears on the display as a fairly wide space between the initial pulse and the front surface reflection because of the reduced velocity of sound in water. The test procedure is given in the applicable specification.

Variations of Immersion Testing

Any one of three techniques may be used in the immersion testing method.

1. The immersion technique, where both the transducer and the test object are immersed in water.
2. The bubbler or squirter technique, where the sound beam is transmitted through a column of flowing water.
3. The wheel transducer technique, where the transducer is mounted in the axle of a liquid filled tire that rolls on the test surface.

In all three of these techniques, a focused transducer that concentrates the sound beam (much like light beams are concentrated when passed through a magnifying glass) may be used to enhance the test. The bubbler and wheel transducer techniques are shown in Figure 5.6

Figure 5.6: Bubbler and wheel transducer techniques.

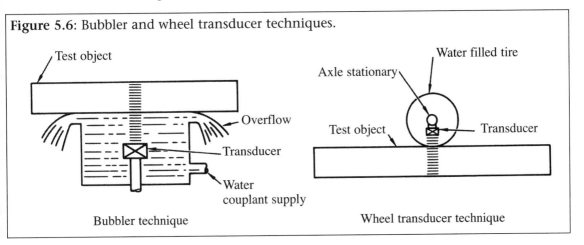

Standard Immersion Technique

In immersion testing, both the transducer and the test object are immersed in water. The sound beam is directed through the water into the material, using either longitudinal waves or shear waves. In many automatic scanning operations, focused beams are used to detect near surface discontinuities or to define minute discontinuities with the concentrated sound beam.

In immersion testing, longitudinal wave transducers are used to accomplish both longitudinal and shear wave testing of the submerged test object. The entry angle of the ultrasonic wave is adjusted manually or by computer setting to produce the precise angle of wave travel (refraction) through the material that will result in a thorough test for anticipated discontinuity orientations. Figure 5.7 shows a typical immersion setup, along with a representation of the display that may be expected in a longitudinal wave examination.

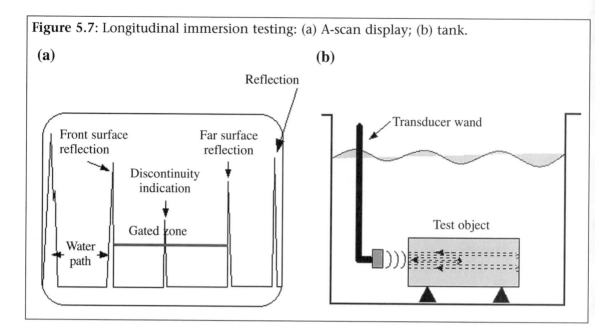

Figure 5.7: Longitudinal immersion testing: (a) A-scan display; (b) tank.

The correct water path distance is particularly important when the test area shown on the A-scan display is gated for automatic signaling and recording operations. The water path distance is carefully set to clear the test area of unwanted signals, such as the second reflection from the front surface, which could cause misinterpretation.

Bubbler Technique

The bubbler technique is a variation of the immersion method. The bubbler is typically used with an automated system for high speed scanning of plate, sheet, strip, rail, tubing and other regularly shaped forms. The sound beam is projected into the material through a column of flowing water and is directed perpendicular to the test surface to produce longitudinal waves. It can also be adjusted at an angle to the surface to produce shear waves.

Figure 5.8 illustrates a bubbler system that is used to test sheet metal moving over a fixed transducer station at high speeds. The same system is also adaptable for use in high speed scanners that can be attached to large immovable objects such as bridge girders or refining industry pressure vessels.

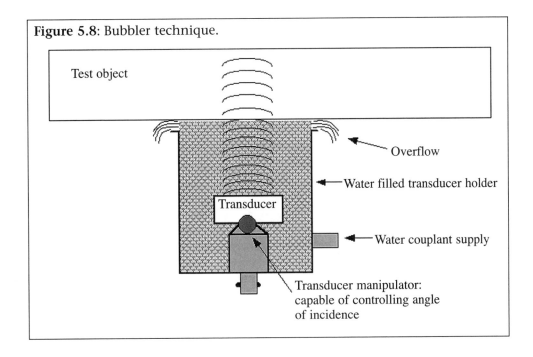

Figure 5.8: Bubbler technique.

Test object

Overflow

Water filled transducer holder

Transducer

Water couplant supply

Transducer manipulator: capable of controlling angle of incidence

Wheel Transducer Technique

The wheel transducer technique is a variant of the immersion method in that the sound beam is projected through a water filled tire into the test object. The transducer, mounted in the wheel axle, is held in a fixed position while the wheel and tire rotate freely. The wheel may be mounted on a mobile apparatus that runs across the material, or it may be mounted on a stationary fixture where the material is moved past it.

It is common practice within the railroad industry to use this ultrasonic testing technique. Wheel mounted transducers are fixed to carriages that are mounted to high rail or rail bound vehicles. Each of the transducer wheels may contain several transducers, and these transducers may be positioned to produce longitudinal and shear tests out of each wheel to detect internal discontinuities within the rails.

Figure 5.9 illustrates the stationary transducer/moving wheel technique. The position and angle of the transducer mounting on the wheel axle may be adjusted to project the desired angle into the test object. The transducer wheel approach provides versatility and efficiency to test personnel within many industrial settings.

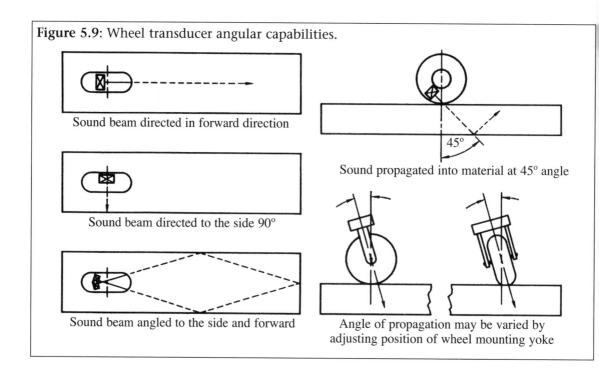

Figure 5.9: Wheel transducer angular capabilities.

Sound beam directed in forward direction

Sound beam directed to the side 90°

Sound beam angled to the side and forward

Sound propagated into material at 45° angle

Angle of propagation may be varied by adjusting position of wheel mounting yoke

AIR COUPLED ULTRASONIC APPLICATIONS

Noncontacting Ultrasonic Techniques

Historically, ultrasonic techniques have required a direct link between the sound source and the test object; that is, a transducer in intimate contact with the test object or coupled by a liquid. In the case of direct contact techniques, this coupling results in transducers being degraded or made ineffective by mechanical wear. Transducer malfunction may also occur with test objects at elevated temperatures. In addition, the requirement for intimate coupling limits inspection flexibility and often calls for elaborate positioning apparatuses to scan an area of interest.

Noncontacting setups have recently been developed. However, the noncontacting feature does not come without certain operational constraints. The most prominent constraint is the drastic decrease in signal strength in comparison to typical piezoelectric transducers.

Table 5.1 summarizes the material characteristics found using laser ultrasonics, electromagnetic acoustic transducers and air coupled transducers to introduce ultrasound into test objects.

Table 5.1. Comparison of noncontact ultrasonic generation and detection techniques.

	Laser ultrasonics	Electromagnetic acoustic transducer	Air coupled transducer
Distance of operation	Large, several meters possible	Millimeters for bulk waves, less for surface, plate or angle beams, performance decreases rapidly with distance	Performance decreases rapidly with distance at 1 MHz and higher, at low frequencies (<50 kHz) many meters of separation is possible
Frequency range	Very large at generation, depends on optical receiver at detection	0.5 to 10 MHz typical	<1 MHz typical, performance decreases rapidly as frequency is increased
Type of waves	Longitudinal, shear vertical, surface, plate	Longitudinal, shear vertical and shear horizontal (both normal to surface and at oblique angles), surface, plate	Longitudinal, (shear vertical, surface, plate by mode conversion)
Orientation	No requirement, sensitivity may decrease at reception away from normal	Should follow the surface	Like conventional transducers
Material	Any, but high laser intensity may damage some materials more than others	Conductive (metals)	Works best with low impedance materials (soft, porous)
Degree of maturity	In development, not yet in industry use	Mature	Mature at low frequencies, in development for frequency >1 MHz
Cost	High (for lasers)	Moderate	Moderate
Safety	May require enclosure or limited access area	No limitation	No limitation
Other features	Operates in vacuum (in space), useful research tool	Operates in vacuum, can control angle of obliquely propagating beams by changing frequency	0.1 to 0.01 atmospheric pressure possible

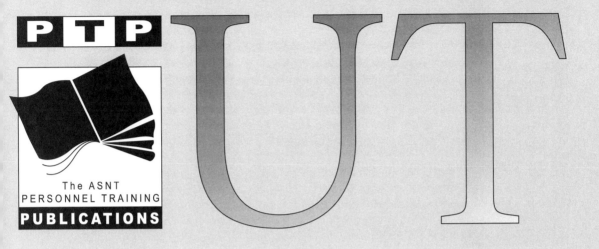

LEVEL II

Chapter 6

Principles of Ultrasonics

REVIEW OF ULTRASONIC TESTING TECHNIQUES

Materials used in the manufacturing of industrial products can sometimes have characteristics that adversely affect the product's intended performance. For example, a small crack in the steel used to build a bridge can grow to a size that reduces the steel's strength to a fraction of what the structure needs for safe operation. As seen in the previous Level I studies, ultrasonic testing is one of the nondestructive testing methods used to detect cracks and other service threatening conditions that can lead to premature failure of critical structures and systems. This chapter reviews the fundamental concepts and various display presentations that allow the ultrasonic technician to investigate and understand the test material, as well as the ultrasonic testing techniques commonly applied in current industrial settings.

FIVE BASIC ELEMENTS OF ULTRASONIC TESTING

Ultrasonic testing is a versatile nondestructive testing method used to detect service threatening conditions in both raw materials and finished products. The test is based on a high frequency mechanical vibration (sound wave) that is made to pass through a test object. To ensure reliable results, the sound wave must be introduced in a consistent and predictable manner. Since high frequency sound waves travel just like the beam of light from a flashlight, the beam can be aimed throughout a test object. Ultrasound is reflected by the boundary between dissimilar materials. For example, sound reflects from a water and solid boundary interface or a boundary between a solid and a gas. Voids or cracks in a material form reflective interfaces.

Unlike light waves, sound waves cannot be seen. The mechanical vibrations used for nondestructive testing are sound waves at a relatively high frequency or pitch. Vibrations with frequencies above our ability to hear them are called *ultrasonic*. For most people, this occurs at frequencies of 20 kHz or higher.

There are five basic elements common to most ultrasonic testing systems.

1. Source of energy.
2. Probing medium.
3. Modifier.
4. Sensitive detector.
5. Display.

Figure 6.1 illustrates an ultrasonic testing system using these five basic elements. The first element is the source of energy that creates the ultrasonic waves. Ultrasonic waves are usually created using transducers that convert electrical pulses into short bursts or pulses of mechanical vibration. Piezoelectricity is a unique material characteristic that converts electrical pulses into ultrasonic pulses, and vice versa. Piezoelectric materials are important components of ultrasonic transducers.

The ultrasonic wave, representing the second element of the test method, is referred to as the *probing medium*. It is used to penetrate test objects in search of clues to the presence of discontinuities or other conditions.

Typical undesirable conditions might include insufficient material thickness, the presence of cracks and voids or poor bonding between layers of laminated structures. These conditions can exist in the raw materials from which an object is made or they may be introduced during a manufacturing process. Service generated factors, such as corrosion, overloading or cyclic stresses, can also degrade the usefulness of a critical test object or assembly.

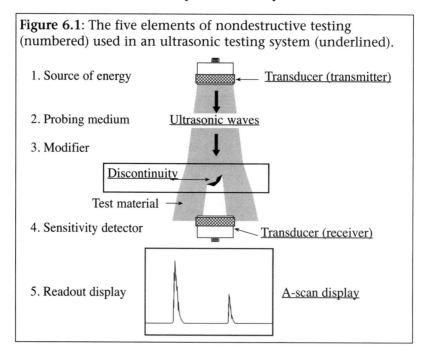

Figure 6.1: The five elements of nondestructive testing (numbered) used in an ultrasonic testing system (underlined).

1. Source of energy   Transducer (transmitter)

2. Probing medium   Ultrasonic waves

3. Modifier

Discontinuity

Test material →

4. Sensitivity detector   Transducer (receiver)

5. Readout display   A-scan display

The third element of ultrasonic testing is some material feature that modifies ultrasonic waves as they pass through the test object. Since ultrasonic waves are mechanical, any change in the mechanical continuity of a test object alters the progress of probing sound waves. A wave can be reflected in a new direction, or, in the case of many small reflectors, it can be scattered into many different directions. For example, a crack in a steel bar represents a very large change in density at the surface of the crack. This is because the density of the air in the crack is much less than the density of the surrounding steel. An ultrasonic wave encountering a crack is totally reflected by the crack's surface.

The fourth element is a sensitive detector capable of registering changes experienced by the probing medium. Such changes can involve wave redirection or unexpected alterations to wave strength. In ultrasonic testing, a transducer is operated as a receiver of ultrasonic pulses and scanned over the external surface of test objects, identifying changes in sound beam direction and pulse strength. Figure 6.2 shows a sound pulse emitted by the source (or sending) transducer. The pulse is detected by another (receiving) transducer when they are positioned face to face on opposite sides of the test object. This configuration, called *through transmission*, is often used to assess the uniformity of test objects throughout their thickness. It is particularly sensitive to the presence of voids, separations and related irregularities found within test materials.

The fifth element of ultrasonic testing is the readout display. Basic ultrasonic testing instruments display the pulses (amplitude and time of arrival) detected by the receiving transducer. More

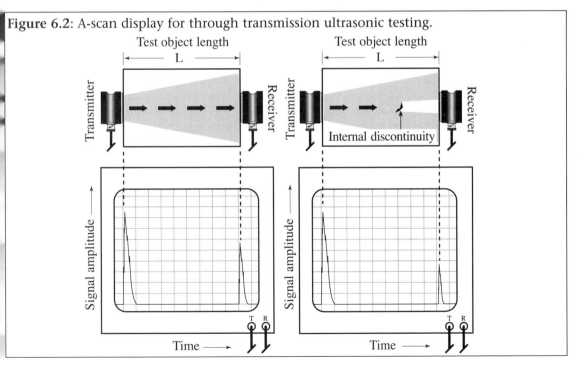

Figure 6.2: A-scan display for through transmission ultrasonic testing.

sophisticated systems gather this same information from many receiver sites and can present graphical displays showing how the acoustic characteristics of the test object vary throughout its cross-section or its entire volume.

ULTRASONIC INSTRUMENTATION

Many configuration variations now exist for ultrasonic testing instrumentation and system hardware. The increasing ability to interface computer capabilities to ultrasonic systems for interpretation, as well as the miniaturization of electrical components, has enlarged the scope of applications for the ultrasonic method.

The ultrasonic testing instrument has three basic functions. The first is to produce an electrical pulse that is used to generate a stress wave in the transducer. The second is to amplify the weak echo signals received from within the test object. The third is to display the returned information in a meaningful way.

Each ultrasonic testing instrument has a pulser, an amplifier and a display device. In order to refresh the information being displayed by the instrument, a system timing circuit is used to repeatedly pulse the transducer and to synchronize the display. Figure 6.3 shows the interconnection of these components along with the connection of a pulse echo transducer (both transmitter and receiver).

Figure 6.3: Components and interconnections of basic discontinuity detector.

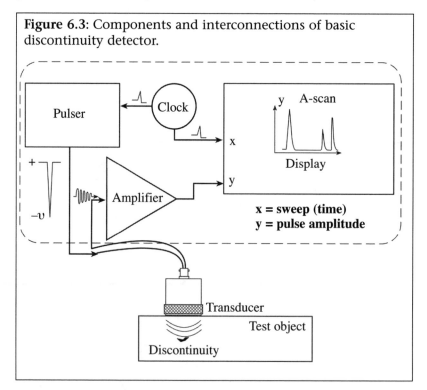

Pulser

When triggered by the clock circuit, most pulsers emit a sharp, unidirectional, spiked pulse that is sent through the coaxial cable to the transducer. In older units using inefficient transducers, this voltage spike might be as much as 1000 V. In newer, digitized instruments with highly efficient transducers and more powerful amplifiers, the excitation voltage may be 200 to 300 V.

In some instruments, the pulser may be adjustable to adapt the instrument to different testing conditions. Lower voltage pulses tend to be shorter, yielding better resolution to signals from closely spaced reflectors. Higher voltages create stronger acoustic pulses that can penetrate to greater depths in highly attenuative materials. To create an electrical match between the pulser circuit and the transducer, supplemental resistance can be used to attain better power transfer. Power transfer is best when the electrical impedance of the transducer matches the output impedance of the pulser circuit.

Certain pulse characteristics can be controlled electronically by the ultrasonic testing instrument. Typically, pulse height (input energy) and duration are adjustable. Although the variability found in an individual ultrasonic testing instrument might be limited, conventional units can be found that generate pulses in the range from 100 V to 1000 V.

The crisp, short duration (single cycle) pulse is used in cases where high resolution of small reflectors is important. The longest pulse is used in cases where penetration is particularly difficult in highly attenuative materials.

The repetition rate at which the pulser is excited is also variable. The pulse repetition rate directly affects the speed at which materials can be tested, particularly in automatic systems. The degree of an object's test coverage can be reduced if the transducer is scanned over a surface at a high speed while the pulse repetition rate is relatively low.

The output pulse is converted to an elastic wave within the transducer. If the transducer is coupled to a test object through a continuous sound path, the wave progresses into the test object. Depending on the test object's acoustic properties (velocity, attenuation and geometry), the stress wave progresses into the material and is reflected at discrete changes in material properties. Depending on reflector orientation and makeup, only part of the stress wave will find its way back to the transducer. After the detected stress wave is reconverted into an electrical signal by the transducer, the magnitude of the pulse will be reduced from the electrical signal used to launch the stress wave.

Amplifier

The *amplifier* of an ultrasonic testing instrument boosts the signal strength of the received pulses to a level that can be easily displayed on the instrument's screen. It is the adjustable gain of the receiver section's amplifier that is the key variable under the control of the technician.

The increase in incoming signal strength can be expressed as a simple linear relationship (relative increase expressed in percentages) or in accordance with a logarithmic relationship (expressed in terms of decibels). Although relative signal strength is a more intuitive means of expressing signal strength (half as large, twice as large, ten times as large), the decibel representations have become most common in ultrasonic testing. A signal level change of 2:1 is expressed as 6 dB. A 2:1 signal loss is –6 dB. A ratio of 100:1 is given as 40 dB, whereas a ratio of 10 000:1 represents an 80 dB gain.

In addition to the relative signal strength, amplifiers can be adjusted to accept either a broad range of signal frequencies or a selected narrower range of frequencies. It serves to filter the echo signals with the purpose of closely amplifying the exact shape of the echo using the broadband setting, or selectively keying in on an individual frequency. When the natural resonance frequency of the transducer matches the narrow band frequency setting, a strong and relatively noise free signal results.

Although the primary purpose of the amplifier component is to increase received signal strength to meet the requirements of the sweep display unit, it is the technician who makes these modifications according to how the echoes appear on the instrument screen. For example, excessively noisy signals can be filtered and clipped by use of controls that act on the amplifier circuit to clean up their appearance. Filtering is used to smooth the jagged appearance of signals while the reject control discriminates against lower strength signals. The result is a clean base line with clearly defined pulse shapes of consistent appearance.

Display Unit

Once the echo signals have been amplified, they are ready to be used in a display mode that gives information about the location and nature of echo surfaces within the test object. Three general formats, A-scan, B-scan and C-scan, are commonly used, with several others incorporated in specific types of equipment.

A-Scan Display

The most common display is called an *A-scan*. In an A-scan display, the vertical axis represents signal strength. The horizontal axis represents time and displays pulse signal amplitude variations with increasing time from a specific reference point. The reference point at the left side of the display screen is usually the moment when the transducer is first excited with an electric pulse, sometimes called the *initial pulse* or *main bang*.

Figure 6.4 shows a typical A-scan presentation. The vertical axis (from 0 to 100 units) reflects the strength or intensity of the mechanical wave activity at the transducer. The horizontal axis (from 0 to 10 units) reflects the sequence of wave activities as a function of elapsed time. Figure 6.4 displays an initial pulse on the left of the screen presentation. The left edge of the pulse corresponds

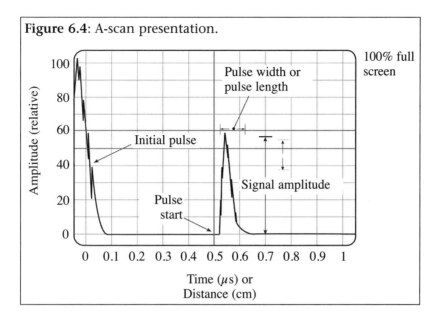

Figure 6.4: A-scan presentation.

to the instant the electrical pulse excited the transducer, while the remainder of the pulse is caused by the ring-down of the transducer.

After a little more than five units of time, an echo stress wave is detected by the transducer. The relative height of the received pulse is a measure of the echo stress wave strength. The horizontal position of the pulse's left edge (labeled *pulse start* in Figure 6.4) is the time the echo pulse arrived at the transducer.

When the signal is displayed, as shown in Figure 6.4, it is correctly called the *video signal*. The bottom horizontal line is often referred to as the *horizontal base line*. Signals from the material cause indications to rise upward from this base line. In this mode, the entire display screen is available for estimating the relative signal's peak amplitude. Note: An alternative A-scan display, called *RF signal*, presents the signal with both positive and negative peaks.

B-Scan Display

The B-scan displays X-positional information in one direction, and the time history of the horizontal scale of the A-scan in the other. The result represents a cross-sectional slice of the reflectors associated with the test object. Figure 6.5 shows the B-scan of a step wedge with internal discontinuities.

Since ultrasound reflects the strongest signal when it encounters a reflector surface at a right angle to its direction of propagation, the B-scan only shows horizontal components of the step wedge and internal reflectors. (Note that the right side of the largest discontinuity on the left is not reflected in the B-scan image because of its orientation compared to the sound beam.) Since internal reflectors reduce the strength of any ongoing ultrasonic waves, a shadow of the internal reflector is often seen as a loss of signal in images of any subsequent reflecting surfaces. Thus, gaps appear in the continuity of the lines representing the wedge step surfaces.

A series of B-scans taken with vertical orientations can be used to build up a three-dimensional image. In practical applications, a particular region within a test object is usually of interest. Often, a single slice is sufficient to gather the information for determining a reflector's location, general size and shape.

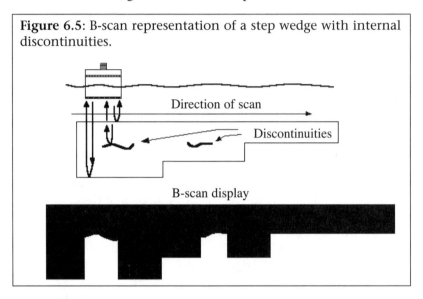

Figure 6.5: B-scan representation of a step wedge with internal discontinuities.

Direction of scan

Discontinuities

B-scan display

C-Scan Display

With a C-scan display, the transducer is scanned in a regular pattern over an area of interest, often using an automatic mechanical positioning device. The received signals are converted to variations in color or grayscale density. Created using A-scan data, the plan view of the test object is generated using signal criteria based on pulse height and time of arrival to determine color or grayscale density at each X and Y location. This is like the floor plan of a house in that the vertical and horizontal directions represent the directions over which the transducer was scanned.

The resulting patterns tend to be directly correlated with the size and shape of the reflecting surfaces within the test object, and therefore are intuitively easy to interpret, like X-ray images. Figure 6.6a shows a C-scan of a test object, indicating the portion of internal reflectors whose signal strength exceeds a predetermined threshold level. The image shows the general shape of the reflector.

For reflectors with sharply defined edges, the image is an accurate representation of the reflector size. A key measure of a C-scan is its ability to distinguish between closely spaced reflectors that exist at the same depth. In this case, the lateral resolution of the system is important and is related to the diameter of the sound beam at the depth of interest, and the scanning step size.

Figure 6.6b shows a C-scan of a test object, using the variations in received signal strength to vary the density of a grayscale (or color ranges for multiple color systems). In this mode, the gradient or rate of signal change is directly related to the rate at which the density or color changes. For a coarse increment between levels, the images can be made to look very similar to contour maps.

Figure 6.6: C-scan renditions of internal discontinuities in test plates: (a) threshold image; (b) contour image; and (c) system layout.

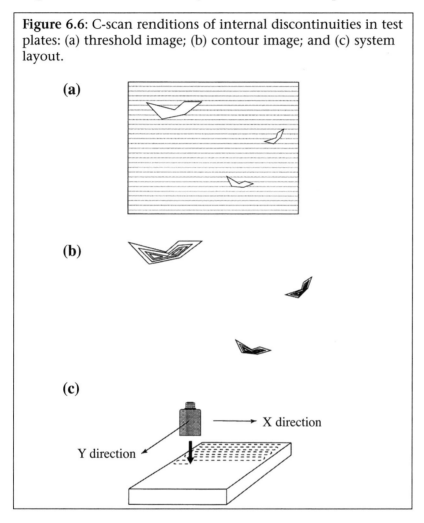

The major advantage of the C-scan representation is the intuitive information related to shape factors that are not readily seen when looking exclusively at the system's A-scan. When the images are created with rather narrow acceptance ranges and carefully correlated with depth information, the C-scan rendition becomes a slice of a three dimensional rendering of the reflectors contained within the test object.

Computerized Systems

The devices used to display the various scan modes can be based on analog or digital technologies. Older instruments are purely analog and have traditionally been equipped with a cathode ray tube to display A-scans. These systems tend to be more bulky and heavier than their newer digital counterparts. However, they reproduce analog signals generated by ultrasonic transducers with very high fidelity and a virtually instantaneous response. They are relatively simple systems, designed to display time varying signals. Their pulse repetition rates or screen replenish rates can be 1000 times per second or more.

Digital devices transform the analog signal into its digital equivalent using an analog-to-digital converter circuit. This process, plus the inherent delay in replenishing screen displays, results in a slower response time for digital systems. Typical computer screens are replenished at a rate of 60 frames per second, a much slower rate of updating the screen presentation. However, because of their small size, digital systems can be equipped with auxiliary features, such as automatic calibration, data storage and external communication, which enhance their functionality well beyond that of analog systems. These features, plus smaller size and weight, facilitate better tests, especially in the application of manual ultrasonic tests.

TRANSDUCERS

All parts of an ultrasonic test system – the instrument, the coupling agent and even the relatively simple coaxial cable – are important in producing a comprehensive inspection of the test object. However, of all the significant advances produced since the 1930s by the scientists and manufacturers of ultrasonic equipment, none have been more important than the improvements made in the manufacture of transducers.

Transducers form the core of all nondestructive ultrasonic testing procedures. Whether an object can be tested or not depends on the appropriate acoustic properties of a transducer. The choice of the correct transducer is decisive for the quality and the reliability of test results.

A transducer is specified for a given test based on its ability to produce a beam of ultrasonic energy. This beam must be capable of penetrating the test object to a calibration standard (representative of the test material) to prescribed depths, and producing reflections that are clearly discernable from fabricated reflectors of prescribed size. Whether the transducer meets the specification will depend on its frequency and its construction.

A transducer's frequency is determined by the thickness of the piezoelectric element (crystal). The thinner the crystal, the higher the frequency. Higher frequency sound beams produce higher levels of sensitivity and resolution, but less ability to penetrate test objects to great depths.

Penetration versus Sensitivity and Resolution

Typically, a transducer is chosen to enhance the sensitivity and the resolution of the system, or to provide for greater ability to penetrate coarse grained materials or test objects of great depths. To gain good penetrating ability, a transducer in the lower frequency range (less than 5 MHz) is used. The lower frequency ranges produce longer wavelengths that counter the natural attenuation of the test material. On the other hand, higher sensitivity to smaller reflectors and better resolution is achieved with higher frequencies (5 MHz and higher).

Transducer Damping

Transducer damping contributes greatly to its characteristic ability of improved penetration or improved sensitivity and resolution. In applications where good resolution is of primary importance, it is common to select a highly dampened transducer. A high degree of damping will help to shorten interface ring-down or recovery time, and allows the system to resolve closely positioned reflectors.

The summaries that follow provide a general impression of the performance characteristics of each transducer type. The technician should remember that each application is unique and requires careful evaluation.

High Penetration: Low Resolution Transducers

Low resolution transducers are intended to provide excellent sensitivity in situations where distance resolution is not of primary importance. Typically, these transducers will have longer waveform duration and a relatively narrow bandwidth.

Medium Penetration: High Resolution Transducers

High resolution transducers are manufactured to reduce the excitation pulse and interface echo recovery time while maintaining good sensitivity at the transducer center frequency.

Broadband Transducers

Broadband transducers are untuned transducers that provide heavily damped broadband performance. They are the best choice in many applications where good axial or distance resolution is necessary. They also serve in tests that require an improved signal-to-noise ratio in coarse grained, attenuating materials.

Test and Documentation

Transducer manufacturers have long acknowledged that transducers, even those manufactured by the same makers to be the same size, shape and frequency, can be highly individual. There is a need for carefully testing and documenting these individual characteristics of ultrasonic transducers.

Today's manufacturers typically provide documentation of the transducer's actual radio frequency waveform and frequency spectrum. Additionally, measurements of peak and center frequency, upper and lower (–6 dB) frequencies, bandwidth and waveform duration are made according to the American Society for Testing and Materials standard *ASTM E-1065*, and are tabulated on a test form and included as part of the purchase of any transducer.

Piezoelectric Materials

The sound beam characteristics of a transducer applied under normal testing conditions are generally derived from the diameter and the frequency of the piezoelectric element. In addition, while the technician knows these features of a given transducer, the details regarding the physical and acoustic properties of the piezoelectric material used to manufacture the actual crystal within the transducer may be unknown. However, this knowledge is important. The material that the crystal is made from determines the efficiency of the overall piezoelectric process, and has an important effect on the overall quality of the ultrasonic test.

The materials from the early days of ultrasonic technology, such as quartz, lithium sulfate or barium titanate, are almost never used today. Instead, new powerful piezoelectric materials are available, but their basic acoustic and electric characteristics are very different. Depending on the application, one material may be more advantageous because of physical or economic reasons, or simply because of a less complicated manufacturing process.

Lead zirconate titanate is the most familiar piezoelectric material used to generate ultrasound. Lead titanate and lead metaniobate are two of today's more frequently used ceramic piezoelectric materials. Manufacturers are also showing rapid progress in their ability to produce composite piezoelectric elements that produce improved signal-to-noise ratios.

TESTING TECHNIQUES

Ultrasonic Testing in Industrial Settings

Ultrasonic testing is used throughout the original manufacturing process and again as a tool for assessing the integrity of components during their useful lifetime. During new component or system manufacturing, ultrasonic testing is used to determine the integrity of basic materials and to monitor fabrication processes, including joining and forming of components. As is the case with most nondestructive testing methods, ultrasonic testing is best used in the early stages of manufacturing when test object geometry is simple.

During their useful lifetime, components and systems are monitored for progressive degradation caused by unexpected overloading, cyclic fatigue cracking, corrosion or environmental conditions. The capacity to monitor the integrity of material from early in the manufacturing process to the very end of a structure's useful life is unique to the application of nondestructive testing in general and ultrasonic testing in particular. For that reason, ultrasonic testing applications are made throughout the maintenance programs of operating power stations, aircraft, petrochemical plants and transportation facilities. Ultrasonic tests ensure that components and systems have been constructed in accordance with original design specifications and that they continue to meet inservice performance projections.

Acoustic Coupling

Unlike light, which can travel through a vacuum, ultrasonic waves require an intermediate medium to transfer the transducer's mechanical motion to the test object. The coupling of the transducer crystal's motion to the test object is best done if the two are rigidly attached to each other, but this is often not possible. If a gas, such as air, is trapped between the transducer and the test object, virtually all the sound energy is reflected at the transducer and air boundary and very little reaches the test object. A liquid couplant is used as a transition medium between the two solid bodies to allow for ease of transducer movement and to displace any air between the transducer and the test object.

In contact testing, the transducer is in direct physical contact with the test object. Successful acoustic wave transfer is best performed when a thin layer of couplant is applied between the transducer and the test object, as shown in Figure 6.7. This couplant ensures effective acoustic energy transfer while lubricating the sliding surfaces between the transducer and the test object.

Figure 6.7: Acoustic couplant – transducer to test object.

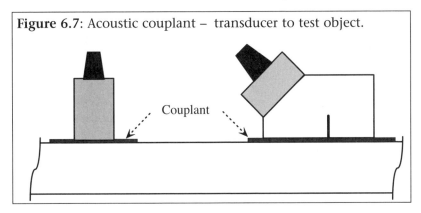

Couplant

Many angle beam transducer-wedge combinations permit the transducer to be attached to the wedge be small screws or a spring-like snap ring. The wedge can be changed to allow the use of other wedge angles and permits combinations of various frequency transducers and angles at minimum cost. When this type of transducer-wedge combination is used, there is also a need to have couplant between the face of the transducer and the wedge, as shown in Figure 6.8. This couplant should be of high viscosity and of a type that does not rapidly evaporate or dry out. Loss of couplant at this point reduces the amount of sound being transmitted into the test object. If the loss occurs after calibration, the result is lower amplitude signals than were used during calibration.

To determine if the transducer is fully coupled to the wedge, the technician should invert the probe, wet the scanning surface then look up the sound path toward the face of the transducer. If the crystal face is completely black, as shown in Figure 6.8a, the transducer is properly coupled. If there are air gaps in the couplant, the crystal face will appear silver-colored or will have areas that are silver-colored, as shown in Figure 6.8b. This indicates that there are air gaps in the couplant. If air gaps are present, the transducer must be recoupled to the wedge and the calibration checked.

Figure 6.8: Acoustic couplant – transducer to wedge.

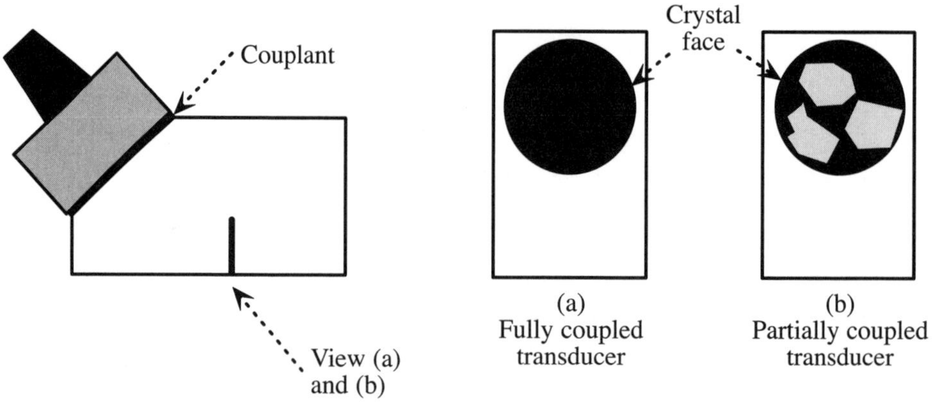

Couplant

View (a) and (b)

Crystal face

(a)
Fully coupled transducer

(b)
Partially coupled transducer

Air Coupling

Spurred by the need to perform some tests without the use of any liquid coming in contact with the test object, dry coupling has been achieved with special synthetic rubber cover materials placed between the transducer and the test object. This approach allows spot tests of objects that are subject to chemical contamination by any form of liquid.

Air coupled transducers can be configured to work in through transmission, like water coupled transducers. It is, however, a distinct feature of air coupled transducers, usually in the 200 to 400 kHz frequency range, to be able to efficiently generate guided plate waves, which are otherwise rapidly dampened by the water couplant. Plate waves generated in such a manner are used today in the testing of many materials and structures. This is particularly the case when testing honeycomb structures. Figure 6.9 illustrates several configurations used to generate guided plate waves within test materials such as plate and tubing.

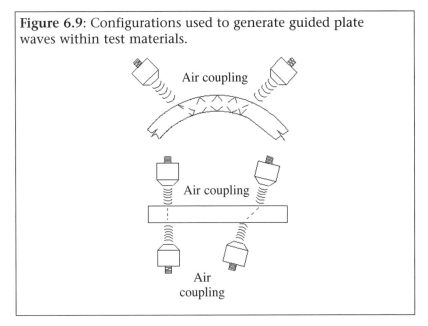

Figure 6.9: Configurations used to generate guided plate waves within test materials.

Typical tests for air coupled transducers include the following.

1. Honeycombs.
2. Solar panels.
3. Foam sandwich panels.
4. Cork coated honeycombs.
5. Aircraft brake disks.
6. Timber and wood products.

It is the combination of specially designed transducers with the proper driver/receiver instrumentation that has made air coupled ultrasonic testing a valuable new tool for industrial ultrasonic testing. Air coupled ultrasonic scanning is increasingly becoming the method of choice for those parts where water and other couplants are not practical.

Immersion Coupling

With immersion coupling, the transducer is somewhat removed from the test object's surface, ensuring continuity of the sound entering the test object by use of an intervening water path. The test object can be immersed within a tank of water, or the water can be introduced along a column between the transducer and the test object surface. Immersion coupling is most often used in automatic scanning applications because of its consistent coupling and the absence of transducer surface wear. Figure 6.10 illustrates a typical immersion setup.

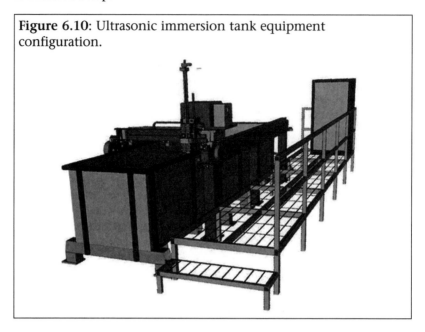

Figure 6.10: Ultrasonic immersion tank equipment configuration.

Immersion systems are widely used in the metal manufacturing industries for offline tests of billets, bars and plates. They are also used for fabricated parts, such as jet engine turbine blades. These systems can be very large, but they are also commonly used on a much smaller scale for laboratory tests and for research and development.

Squirter Systems

Another form of immersion testing is known as the *squirter system*. As shown in Figure 6.11, the system is most often used with transducers aiming their pulsed or continuous wave beams through water columns that carry the beams to the surface of the test object. Squirter systems are used to test composite materials in aerospace manufacturing. These systems can be very large and complex. For example, systems greater than 40 ft long are quite common, although much smaller systems are also manufactured.

Figure 6.11: Ultrasonic testing by use of water columns, known as the *squirter system*.

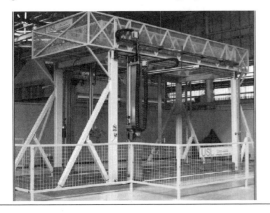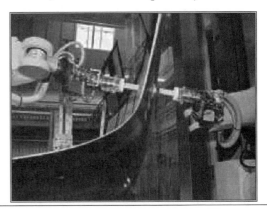

BASE MATERIAL TESTING

The straight beam testing of base materials involves directing the sound beam through the test object perpendicular to the scanning surface. Since the sound beam travels through thickness, most test objects can be tested from one side. The transducer should be moved across the surface, as shown in Figure 6.12 so that each successive pass overlaps the previous scan. The amount of overlap is usually defined in the governing code or specification.

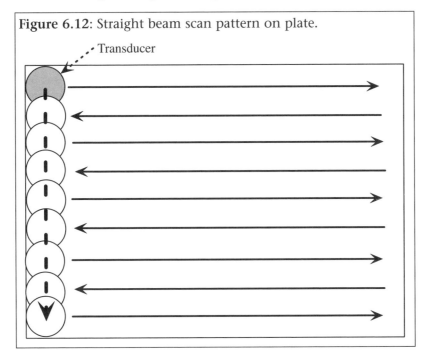

Figure 6.12: Straight beam scan pattern on plate.

Transducer

On large plate, it is common to perform straight beam tests using a grid pattern of scanning. The grid is laid out in accordance with the governing code or specification, and the transducer is moved along those grid lines. If a discontinuity is found, the test is concentrated in that area until the full area of the discontinuity has been outlined and marked on the surface of the test object.

When performing angle beam tests on plate, a full test will require scans in four directions to detect discontinuities aligned both parallel and perpendicular to the rolling direction, as shown in Figure 6.13. Scanning in opposing directions in both the axial and transverse directions will detect skewed discontinuities that might not be oriented perpendicular to the sound beam in one direction.

Figure 6.13: Angle beam scan patterns for plate.

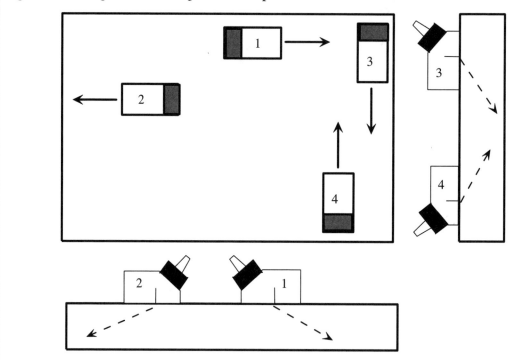

Angle beam testing of pipe is performed in a similar manner, with two scans around the circumference in opposite directions and in two opposing directions parallel to the axis of the pipe. On the circumferential scans, a wedge specifically contoured to match the pipe's outer diameter is usually required.

Weld Testing
Straight beam testing of welds can only be performed on welds that have had the weld reinforcement ground flush or from the back side of tee or corner welds, and then only if permitted by the governing code or specification.

Angle beam testing can be performed on full penetration plate butt welds, corner and tee welds and pipe welds. The first step in the testing process is to determine the accessibility to the area of interest. Many codes and specifications require ultrasonic testing of the base material scanning surface beyond the toe of the weld which is done as described previously. The available distance back from the weld should be taken into consideration when selecting a wedge angle and determining the length of the scanning area.

Figure 6.14 shows three common weld configurations: butt welds in a plate, a corner joint made by two plate ends set at 90° angles to each other, and a tee joint between two plates (as typically seen in a structural beam-column connection). The surfaces adjacent to, or in the case of corner and tee welds, the face directly behind, the weld are the surfaces from which the weld can be ultrasonically scanned. As shown in all three figures, these are commonly labeled faces *A*, *B* and *C*, where applicable.

The two weld sketches in 6.14a show plates with two weld configurations, a single-vee butt weld at the top and a double-vee butt weld at the bottom. While the scanning surfaces for both are labeled the same, the location of the root of the weld is different and will affect the location of certain types of discontinuities. The *A* face is on the plate side with the weld crown for a single-vee weld with the *B* side being on the root side. In the case of a double-vee weld, the *A* face is usually the side of the weld that is most easily accessible.

Figure 6.14b shows a typical corner weld with the *A* scanning surface being on the weld crown side of the beveled plate, the *B* face being the opposite side of the same plate and the *C* face being directly opposite of the beveled plate on the reverse side of the other plate. These face designations are the same for a typical tee-weld, as shown in Figure 6.14c. Scanning from the *C* face is done with a straight beam transducer and is used primarily to detect laminar tears in the vertical member behind the weld or sidewall lack of fusion at the vertical face of the weld groove (as shown). In all tests, the face from which the weld is being tested should be recorded on the test report form.

Once the scanning face has been selected, it is necessary to determine how much of that surface will be required to perform an test that provides full coverage of the area of interest. This is determined by the material thickness and the choice of the wedge angle if that choice is left up to the technician and not specified by the code or specification. In order to attain full volumetric coverage, it is necessary to ensure that the weld area is scanned by both the first and second legs of the sound beam. If an additional portion of the base metal requires testing, that distance must be added to the scanning area.

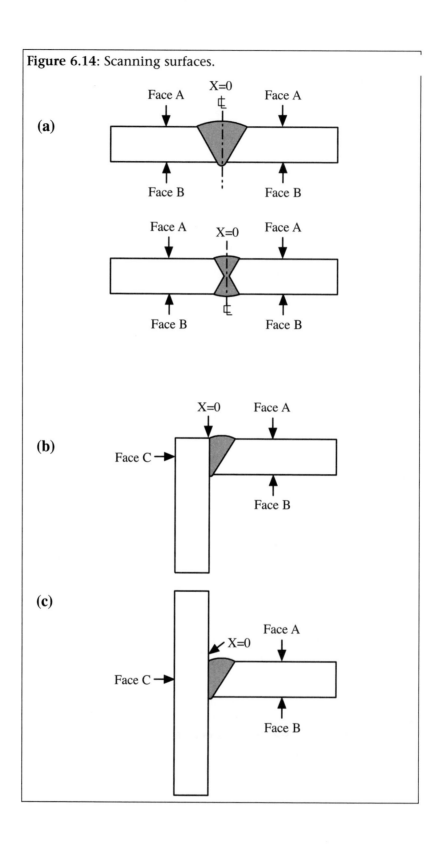

Figure 6.14: Scanning surfaces.

Figure 6.15 shows the minimum scanning distance that will be required on each side of a plate butt weld to provide full coverage of the weld volume. In the figure, the *A* face is the scanning surface and the weld is being scanned from both sides. At position *A1*, where the nose of the transducer hits the edge of the weld crown, the sound beam only covers a small portion of the bottom of the weld. At position *B1*, from the other side of the weld, only an additional small volume that was not covered by *A1* is scanned. However, as the transducer is moved back away from the weld, towards positions *A2* and *B2* respectively, the sound beam will cross the entire cross-section of the weld resulting in full coverage of the weld volume. If the governing documents require that a portion of the base metal also be interrogated, then that distance must also be included when the scanning surface is prepared. Technicians should keep in mind that a 70° transducer will require a much longer scan path than will a 45° probe, but a 45° sound beam may be too short to get the second leg clear through the weld cross-section before the nose of the probe hits the edge of the weld crown.

Figure 6.15: Minimum scanning distance.

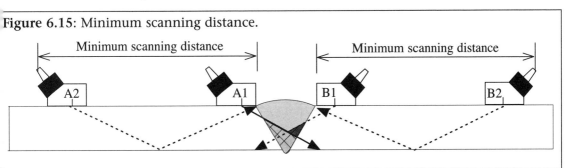

To prepare the scanning surface, that portion of the plate must be free of any loose scale, rust or other foreign material that might cause a bad couple that would prevent the sound from entering the test object. If weld spatter is present, it may be necessary to use a cold chisel to remove it. A 7.6 cm (3 in.) wide chisel is a good tool for this purpose as it is wide enough to clean a large area quickly and if used properly will not gouge the plate surface. Once the scanning surfaces have been prepared, the couplant can be applied and the weld scanned.

In order to detect both transverse and axially oriented discontinuities, the weld has to be scanned in two directions from both sides of the weld. For axial discontinuities (those that run parallel to the weld length) the transducer is aimed at the weld and moved back and forth on side *A* of the plate surface, as shown in Figure 6.16. For transversely oriented discontinuities (those that run across the weld width) the transducer is slid along the side of the weld in both directions, as shown on the *B* surface. Both types of scans are performed from both the *A* and *B* surfaces to ensure that all orientations of discontinuities are found.

Figure 6.16: Angel beam scan patterns for welds.

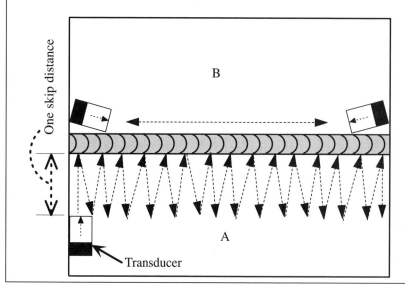

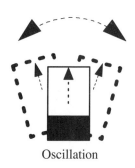

As the probe is moved back and forth, the sound beam is required to overlap the previous scan by some percentage. The scan that is shown on the left side of Figure 6.17 shows a scan pattern using a 50% overlap. If the amount of overlap is not detailed in the governing documents, a 20 to 50% overlap is usually used. The easiest way to estimate the percentage of overlap is to look at the tracks the transducer makes in the couplant on the plate surface.

As the transducer is moved back and forth, it should also be oscillated from side to side in order to detect discontinuities that may not be perfectly oriented at 90° to the sound beam. If no oscillation requirement is specified in the governing code or specification, a range of approximately 15° to 20° can be used, as shown in Figure 6.17.

These manipulations seem to be relatively straight-forward and at first glance do not seem to be a complex tasks. However, all of this needs to be done while the technician is watching the CRT screen, not the probe, and many technicians may routinely use probes varying from 0.64 to 2.5 cm (0.25 to 1 in.) in diameter (or greater) so the difficulty in maintaining a good scanning pattern with a consistent overlap becomes apparent. It is only with practice that this ability is developed.

To further complicate the process, most codes or standards require that the scanning rate not exceed a maximum travel speed. A common restriction is that the scan speed cannot exceed 15 cm (6 in.) per second, though the actual scan speed will either be detailed in the governing specification or in one of the specification's referenced documents. The purpose of this restriction is to ensure that any reflected sound has time to return to the transducer before it has moved on.

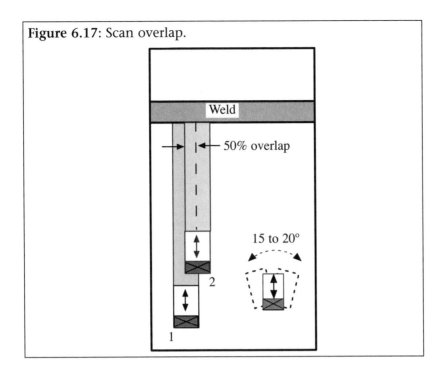

Figure 6.17: Scan overlap.

Weld

50% overlap

15 to 20°

2

1

The final step before beginning the test is to select a set of reference points so that the locations of any discontinuities can be accurately located. To do this, the most common system is to use an X–Y coordinate system, where the X-axis represents the distance across the weld and the Y-axis represents the distance along the length of the weld. The typical locations for these points for the different weld types are shown in Figure 6.18.

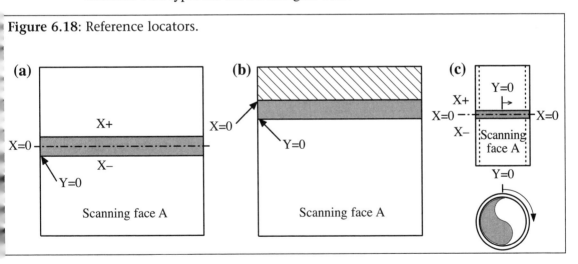

Figure 6.18: Reference locators.

(a)

X+

X=0

X–

Y=0

Scanning face A

(b)

X=0

Y=0

Scanning face A

(c)

X+

X=0

X–

Y=0

X=0

Scanning face A

Y=0

As can be seen in Figure 6.18a, the zero point for X on a plate weld is the centerline of the weld (X=0), and the zero point for Y (Y=0) is the left end of the weld. For corner and tee welds, the X zero point is at the back side of the weld, as shown in Figure 6.18b. For pipe welds 6.18c it is common to place the Y=0 reference point on top of the pipe for horizontal runs and in line with an elbow or fitting on vertical runs. The X=0 point is again the centerline of the weld. However, some codes and specifications do have specific conventions for these locations so they should be checked prior to setting your own locating marks. If no specific location instructions are given, the technician should select one set of conventions and record them on the report form. It is also smart to mark Y=0 on the weld so that if repairs are needed the welder will know where to start measuring from.

The distance of a discontinuity from Y=0 is fairly obvious; the distance is measured from the left end of the weld to the nearest end of a discontinuity. Therefore, a discontinuity that starts at 15 cm (6 in.) from the left end of the weld and ends 20 cm (8 in.) from the left end would be listed as a 5 cm (2 in.) indication at Y=15 cm (Y=6 in.).

To locate a discontinuity on the X axis requires a little more thought. Centerline indications are easy; they're at X=0, as shown by indication *A* on the shaded weld shown in Figure 6.19. Discontinuity *B* is 1.3 cm (0.5 in.) from the centerline *away* from the technician, and would be recorded as being at X=+1.3 cm (X=+0.5 in.). Because *C* and *D* indications are both on the near side of X=0, they would be recorded as being at X=−1.3 cm (X=−0.5 in.) and X=−0.6 cm (X=−0.25 in.), respectively. When scanning the weld from the other side, the technician should make sure that the X+ and X− convention are not accidentally reversed.

Figure 6.19: X-axis locations +/−.

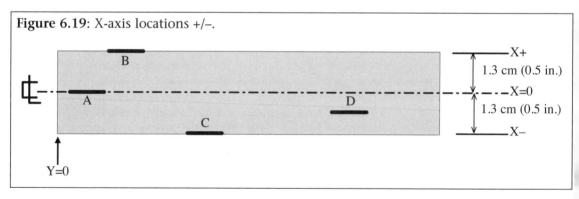

When sizing a discontinuity for length, the technician should refer to the governing documents for direction. However, if a specific method of determining the end point is not given, it is common practice to use the 6 dB drop method for making that determination. If used, that fact should be recorded. The 6 dB drop method refers to the fact that a decrease of 6 dB of gain will result in a decrease in screen amplitude of 50%. The technician will manipulate the transducer to maximize the signal from an indication.

Once that is done, the maximized signal is set to 80% full screen height (FSH), as shown in Figure 6.20a. The transducer is then slowly moved to the left parallel to the axis of the discontinuity until the screen signal drops to 40% full screen height, or 50% of the maximized signal (a 6dB drop) as shown in Figure 6.20b. A mark is then made on the plate surface at the centerline of the transducer to denote that end of the discontinuity. The transducer is then moved back toward the other end of the discontinuity until the signal peaks at 80% full screen height and again drops to 40% at the other end of the indication, as shown in Figure 6.20c. This end is marked using the centerline of the transducer as before and the distance between the two marks is recorded as the length of the discontinuity.

Figure 6.20: Sizing using 6 dB drop.

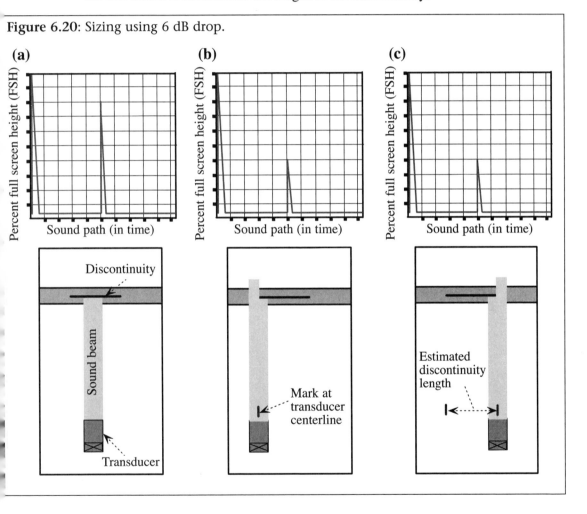

Since many discontinuities are irregular in shape, the technician should continue the sizing scan past the point at which a 50% amplitude drop is first seen. It is entirely possible that a discontinuity will have a varying orientation that will drop off in amplitude at one point then increase in amplitude again farther away from the center of the discontinuity. If this condition occurs and the scan is stopped when the signal first drops to 50%, the recorded length will not reflect the actual discontinuity length. If the acceptance-rejection criterion being used is based on a combination of length and decibel rating, miscalculation of the length could have serious results.

The depth of a discontinuity can also be calculated using a trigonometric function based on the sound path or surface distance and the test angle; it can be read directly from a graphic ultrasonic testing calculator, or with the newer machines, it can be automatically calculated by pushing a button. However, regardless of how the depth is calculated, the technician should bear in mind that the depth calculation is based on the nominal wedge angle (45°, 60° or 70°), and most codes and specifications allow the transducer to vary within a range of +/–2°. As a result, a three decimal place (0.002 cm [0.001 in.]) depth may not be as accurate as the technician might think.

Chapter 7

Equipment Calibration

INTRODUCTION

The equipment used in ultrasonic testing involves electronic and mechanical devices working together to accurately capture the way ultrasonic waves interact with various features of test materials. Ultrasound interaction within a given material is analyzed by measuring the strength and the nature of returning waves. Location of reflectors is deduced by knowing the direction of the wave's propagation and the time elapsed in the wave's travel from the sending source to the receiving device. The speed of sound in the test object must be known for accurate distance estimations. For simple test object geometries such as plate materials, the ultrasonic testing instrument can be used to interpret features such as thickness and presence of major discontinuities. As the geometric complexity of test objects increases, interpretation of detected ultrasonic wave signals becomes more difficult. To interpret results precisely, the fundamental characteristics of the ultrasonic testing system must be known.

Equipment calibration is the process of repeatedly verifying that the ultrasonic equipment is performing as intended. It is carried out at the transducer level, the instrument level and the integrated system level. The frequency of calibration is based on practical field experience and is often mandated through consensus codes and standards.

Transducers are usually checked for their general condition and conformance to specified performance criteria, such as beam angle, depth resolution and absence of excessive reverberation noise, before beginning tests. The instrument's general condition is also checked. An ultrasonic test system's conformance to linearity performance limits is occasionally checked in a calibration laboratory, however, it is routinely adjusted to meet specific amplitude and distance calibration criteria before each field test. Finally, the transducer instrument positioning system is monitored for ongoing conformance to settings established at the beginning of each test. The frequency of system checks is usually mandated by test procedure specification, and is based on the risks of losing valid test data caused by the system falling out of calibration.

This chapter discusses how transducers, ultrasonic testing instruments and overall testing systems are calibrated during normal test practices.

TRANSDUCER PERFORMANCE CHECKS

In general, the performance characteristics of transducers can be measured as they relate to fundamental generation and reception of ultrasonic energy or as part of checking their practical behavior related to testing effectiveness. The former is typically done in a laboratory equipped with special testing and positioning apparatuses. The latter is done by the technician before, during and after routine field tests.

Considered as a stand alone component, transducers can be characterized by their electrical and acoustic responses. Typical features include electrical amplitude and frequency responses, such as relative pulse echo sensitivity, center frequency, frequency bandwidth, time response, electrical impedance and sound field measurements. Typical approaches to transducer characterization can be found in documents such as the *Standard Guide for Evaluating Characteristics of Ultrasonic Search Units, ASTM E-1065.*

Transducers designed to generate angled shear waves are checked for depth resolution, precise beam location and refraction angle within a specified material. A standard widely used for this purpose is the International Institute of Welding calibration block (the *IIW block*).

INSTRUMENT CALIBRATION

Amplitude Linearity

In analog instruments, measurements of signal strength (pulse height) and transit time (related to distance from sending transducer) are taken directly from the display screen. It is important in these instruments that the visual A-scan axes be directly proportional to incoming signal strength (vertical axis) and expended time (horizontal axis). Both axes must remain linear with respect to these two incoming signals throughout the operating range of the instrument. Since these variables are exclusively in the domain of the instrument's electronic circuitry, their calibration for linearity is often performed by technicians familiar with electronic circuitry during routine maintenance in the laboratory.

On-site checks of amplitude linearity (vertical axes) can be performed by observing how pairs of pulses, which differ in amplitude by some fixed amount, maintain their relative amplitude difference while changing the instrument's amplification. If the amplifier is linear, the ratio of the two pulses will remain the same as the gain of the instrument is changed over its operational range. An example of this is shown in Figure 7.1, where two signals are set to 80% and 40% of full screen height (FSH) in Figure 7.1a. The gain setting is then decreased by 6 dB, which should decrease the signal amplitudes by 50% resulting in the signals dropping to 40% and

20% FSH respectively, as shown in Figure 7.1b. If similar checks across the full vertical range (0 to 100% FSH) are within tolerance, the machine is considered to be linear in the vertical direction. Tolerances can be found in *ASTM E-317*, Figure 3.

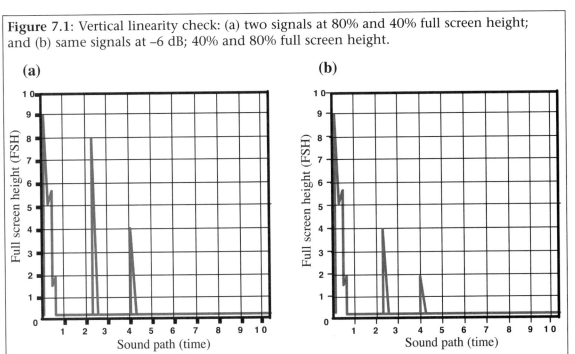

Figure 7.1: Vertical linearity check: (a) two signals at 80% and 40% full screen height; and (b) same signals at –6 dB; 40% and 80% full screen height.

The basic calibration steps before a test include establishing the horizontal axis scale to correspond to the physical region of interest within the test object, and setting a basic sensitivity level (based on a standard reflector). When tests are made over extensive sound travel paths, assessments of effective sound attenuation are also taken and included in the calibration process. When test objects have contours and surface conditions different from those of the calibration block, these differences need to be assessed and compensations made when interpreting test results.

STRAIGHT BEAM CALIBRATION

For a simple longitudinal wave transducer (straight beam) test instrument, system level calibration typically uses any calibration block with a known thickness or depth to establish the range of thickness directly displayed on the screen. Using the multiple echoes as a relative gage, the screen width can be set to represent any distance significant to the test. Figure 7.2 shows a linear screen capable of displaying echoes at depths up to 13 cm (5 in.).

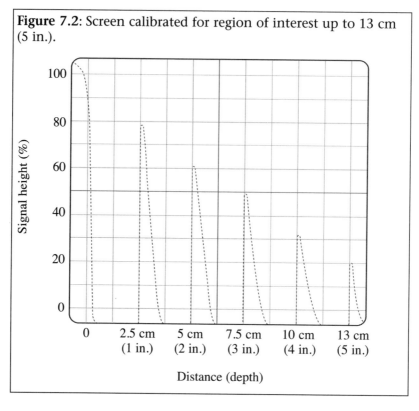

Figure 7.2: Screen calibrated for region of interest up to 13 cm (5 in.).

The sensitivity of the system is adjusted based on a standard reference reflector. Both side drilled holes (SDHs) and flat bottomed holes (FBHs) are used for this purpose. In special cases, custom reflectors placed in test object mockups are used to simulate the actual condition and testing environments of specific critical components.

Flat bottomed holes have historically been used as the basis for calibrating straight beam testing systems. Calibration blocks, called *area amplitude blocks*, are available in sets with a range of hole sizes. This allows setting basic sensitivities for relatively large reflectors (low sensitivity) through very small reflectors (requiring a highly sensitive detection system). Typical area amplitude blocks have FBH diameters that range from 1/64 to 8/64 in. (0.038 to 0.317 cm [0.015 to 0.125 in.]).

With area amplitude blocks, the sound path remains constant and the hole diameter changes. As a result of the reduced FBH surface area seen by the sound beam, the amplitude decreases as the FBH diameter decreases (amplitudes *A*, *B* and *C* on the screen representation in Figure 7.3). However, the location of the screen signal does not change horizontally since the sound path remains constant. A representation of this (not to scale) is shown in Figure 7.3.

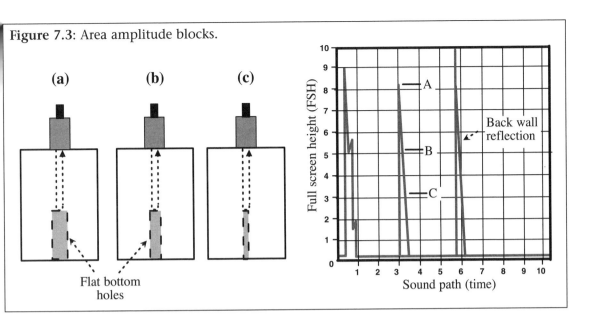

Figure 7.3: Area amplitude blocks.

(a) (b) (c)

Flat bottom holes

Full screen height (FSH)

A

B

C

Back wall reflection

Sound path (time)

When the region to be tested involves relatively thick sections, the calibration process needs to determine the effective drop in sound energy with increasing distance. For straight beam applications, this is often done using distance amplitude blocks. These sets of blocks typically have FBHs of the same diameter, usually 3/64, 5/64 or 7/64 in. (0.13, 0.2 or 0.28 cm [0.05, 0.08 or 0.11 in.]). Each set of blocks come with sound path distances ranging from 1.6 to 14.6 cm (0.625 to 5.75 in.). They are used sequentially to establish the pattern of changes in reflector echo signal strength with increasing distance from the transducer. Figure 7.4 shows a general representation of three distance amplitude blocks and a typical screen presentation for each block.

Note that the decrease in screen amplitude is due to the increasing length of the sound path, not a change in FBH diameter. Unlike the area amplitude blocks, the signal location moves horizontally to the right as the sound path increases. The loss in amplitude is due to beam spread and attenuation that results in less of the sound beam seeing the FBH. If a curve were drawn from the peaks of each signal, that curve would be called a *distance amplitude correction (DAC) curve*. Figure 7.5 shows a typical pattern called a distance amplitude correction curve for a 13-block set.

The response curve derived from the distance amplitude holes becomes the basis for correcting readings taken during actual tests. For example, a discontinuity at a depth of 5 cm (2 in.), with the same effective reflecting area as another at a depth of 10 cm (4 in.), will appear on the screen to be four times bigger than the deeper reflector.

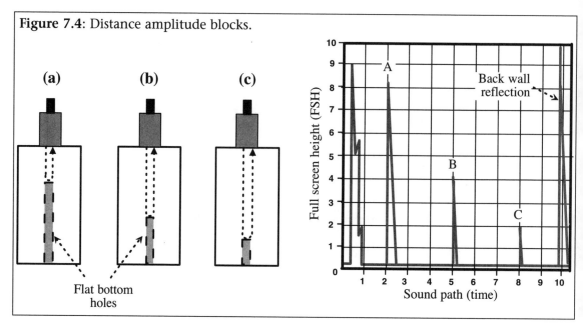

Figure 7.4: Distance amplitude blocks.

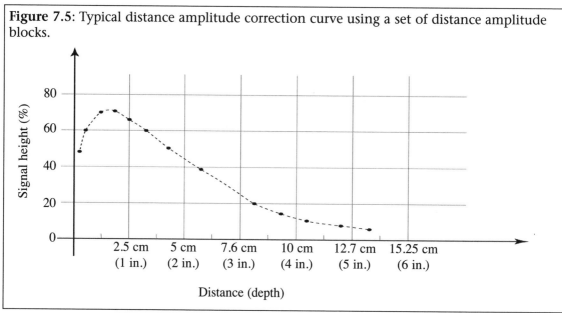

Figure 7.5: Typical distance amplitude correction curve using a set of distance amplitude blocks.

When using calibration blocks for ultrasonic testing, the required sensitivity is based on the size of the reference reflector, typically a flat bottomed hole or a side drilled hole. For tests with longer sound paths, the attenuation of the sound is estimated by creation of an appropriate distance amplitude correction curve. Additional corrections used to compensate for surface curvature, roughness or differences in the acoustic properties of the block and test object may also be required in special cases. Some of these cases are discussed in the context of certain standards covered in Chapter 11.

ANGLE BEAM CALIBRATION

Side drilled holes have traditionally been used as the basis for calibrating angle beam test systems. Calibration blocks with side drilled holes have an added advantage: the amount of sound reflected from a side drilled hole remains the same regardless of the transducer angle. Several of the more common blocks used for angle beam calibration are the basic calibration block, the International Institute of Welding (IIW) block and the distance-sensitivity calibration (DSC) block.

Basic Calibration Block

The basic calibration block, shown in Figure 7.6, is rectangular with varying size and thickness, with thickness selection based on the thickness of the test object. The diameter of the side drilled holes vary based on the thickness; increasing in diameter as the block thickness increases. The holes are drilled and reamed to size so that the inner surface of the holes is as smooth as possible to provide a uniform reflector.

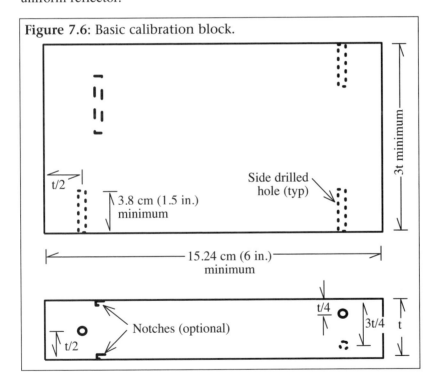

Figure 7.6: Basic calibration block.

The block must be long enough to allow a full skip distance for the transducer that is to be used, but may not be less than 15 cm (6 in.). As the thickness increases, the block will need to be longer to accommodate the longer skip distances.

The most common way to calibrate using the basic calibration block is to use the depth of each hole from the scanning surface to set the screen width. Figure 7.7 shows the sound paths for the first legs for 1/4t, 2/4 (1/2)t and 3/4t hole locations and the corresponding screen locations for each signal. Note that hole depths are designated in 1/4t increments.

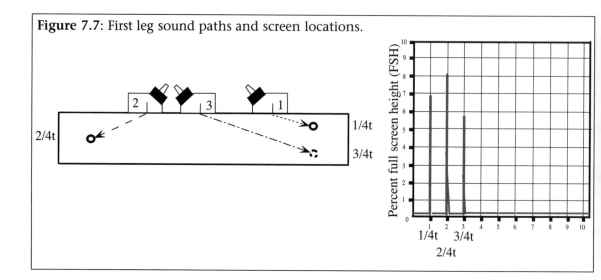

Figure 7.7: First leg sound paths and screen locations.

Figure 7.8 shows the same holes being interrogated in the second leg of the sound beam. Because the backwall of the block would be 1t, or 4/4t, and the sound hits the backwall at an angle, there is no reflection at 4/4t. However, when the 3/4t hole is seen in the second leg, the resulting sound path would be the same as if the hole was 1-1/4t, or 5/4t, below the scanning surface.

This can be seen graphically by imagining a mirror image of the block as shown by the shaded section in Figure 7.8 and imagining the sound path as continuing in a straight line. Similarly, when the 1/2t hole is seen in the second leg, the imaginary depth would be 6/4t and the 1/4t hole would show up at the 7/4t location. The 8/4t depth would be the scanning surface after a full skip distance, and as with the 4/4t depth, no reflection is seen. Because the sound paths are longer than those of the first leg, less sound is reflected and the resulting screen amplitudes are correspondingly lower, as shown.

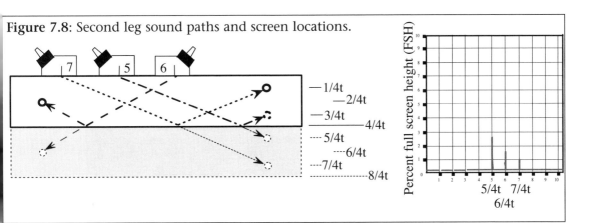

Figure 7.8: Second leg sound paths and screen locations.

Now the use of the depth designation in one-quarter thickness increments becomes apparent. Each one of the depths can be depicted on the screen at the corresponding graticule marker. That is, the 1/4t signal can be set at the first major graticule, the 2/4t signal at 2, etc. By doing this the screen, from zero to the eighth graticule, accurately represents twice the thickness of the calibration block being used.

To begin this type of calibration, the technician should maximize the return signal from the 1/4t hole, set the amplitude to 80% full screen height (FSH), then place it over the first graticule. The transducer is then slid backwards on the block until the 1/4t hole is seen in the second leg (7/4t location). This signal is then placed over the seventh graticule. The transducer is then moved forward again to hit the 1/4t hole in the first leg, and using the range and delay controls and repeating this process, the screen is adjusted until the 1/4t and 7/4t holes line up over the first and seventh graticules, as shown in Figure 7.9.

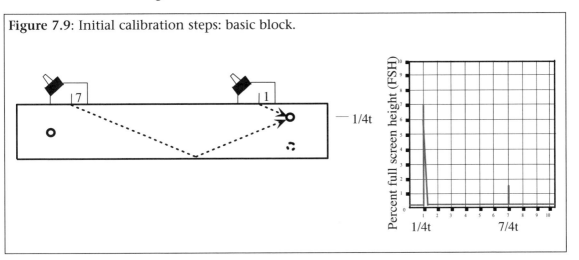

Figure 7.9: Initial calibration steps: basic block.

At this point, the signals from the other four locations (2/4t, 3/4t, 5/4t and 6/4t) should line up over the second, third, fifth and sixth major graticules, respectively. If they do not, the range and delay controls should be adjusted until all signals line up where they belong. As noted previously, there will be no screen signals at the 4/4t and 8/4t locations.

In some instances, the signal amplitude from the 2/4t hole may be higher than the amplitude of the signal from the 1/4t hole. If this occurs, the gain (decibel level) should be set so that the signal from the 2/4t hole is set at 80% FSH (or whatever screen height is specified in the governing code or specification) and the signal locations from all six hole positions should be rechecked. This gain setting should be recorded, as it becomes the reference level for the inspection process.

Without changing the reference level gain setting, the peak of each maximized signal can be marked on the screen using a china marker, and those points can be connected to create a DAC curve similar to that shown in Figure 7.5. This curve, shown in Figure 7.10, then becomes the rejection level for signals found during the test. (Note: Some codes require that a line be marked at 50% DAC height, which is shown by the light dashed line in Figure 7.10). Since there are no signals from the scanning surface at the zero (0) and 8/8t positions, the DAC curve should be extrapolated back to zero and out to the 8/8 screen position.

When inspecting using a DAC curve, scanning is performed at a gain level above the reference level (as described in the governing code or specification) and if an indication is found, the gain is reset to the reference level. If the signal amplitude at reference exceeds DAC, the indication is rejectable.

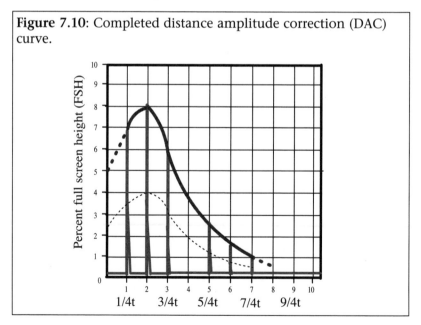

Figure 7.10: Completed distance amplitude correction (DAC) curve.

International Institute of Welding (IIW) Block

Another commonly used calibration block is the International Institute of Welding (IIW) block. This block comes in several different types and in multiple materials. For this discussion, the Type 1 IIW block, shown in Figure 7.11, will be used.

Figure 7.11: Type 1 IIW block.

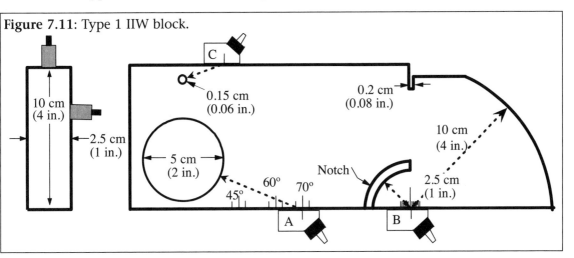

This block provides the technician with many options. For straight beam calibration the block can be scanned from the side (2.5 cm [1 in.] thickness) to set up screen widths in 2.5 cm (1 in.) multiples, or from the edge through the 4 in. width for wider screen widths, and the 0.2 cm (0.08 in.) notch can be viewed from the opposite side of the block to check transducer resolution.

For angle beam work, the angle of the transducer wedge can be placed in position *A* on the IIW block and the return signal from the 5 cm (2 in.) diameter hole maximized. With the signal maximized, the technician can see where the exit point of the wedge is located. In the figure, the transducer exit point is shown on the 70° line, so this transducer wedge angle is within acceptable tolerance. Many codes and specifications require that the actual wedge angle be within +/–2° of the nominal angle (45°, 60° or 70°). If the actual wedge angle is outside of the specified range, the transducer may not be used for inspection work until it is brought back into the acceptable range.

Note: Most wedges can be corrected by sanding the scanning face on a flat surface. For wedges that have a low angle (<68°), the rear of the wedge should be sanded down; for wedges with high angles (>72°), the nose should be sanded down.

Prior to beginning a calibration using the IIW block, the technician must determine what screen width will be required to perform the test. Unlike DAC curve calibrations on a basic block, when the IIW block is used the screen width is not determined by the depth of reference holes. Screen width selection in an IIW calibration is based on the length of the full sound path skip distance in the material to be tested, with the selected screen width sufficiently wide to allow a full skip distance to be completely seen on the screen. However, screen width should not be excessively wide as that can cause signals to display too close to each other on the screen, making it difficult for the technician to discriminate between individual signals.

Two of the most commonly used screen widths are 12.7 cm (5 in.) and 25.4 cm (10 in.) One advantage to using these screen widths is that for the 12.7 cm (5 in.) screen each major graticule along the baseline will be equivalent to 1.27 cm (0.5 in.) of sound path, and on a 25.4 cm (10 in.) screen each major graticule will be equivalent to 2.5 cm (1 in.) of sound path.

To determine the appropriate screen width, the technician should determine which wedge angle is to be used (this may be dictated by the governing code or specification) and the thickness of the material to be tested. The technician then calculates one full skip distance for that material thickness. If the full skip distance is less than 12.7 cm (5 in.), a 12.7 cm (5 in.) screen width should be sufficient. If the full skip distance is greater than 12.7 cm (5 in.), then a wider screen width (such as 25.4 cm [10 in.]) must be used. For example, on a 1.9 cm (0.75 in.) thick test object using a 70° wedge angle, a full skip distance will be approximately 11.7 cm (4.625 in.), so a 12.7 cm (5 in.) screen width can be used. However, on 3.175 cm (1.25 in.) thick material, the full skip distance for a 70° wedge will be approximately 19.4 cm (7.625 in.), so a 25.4 cm (10 in.) screen would be appropriate.

Cautionary note: If the screen width selected is less than a full skip distance, then the far end of the second leg of the sound beam will not show on the screen and the upper portion of the material or weld being tested will not be seen by the technician, invalidating the testing process.

Once the screen width is selected, the transducer is placed at position B on the IIW block as shown in Figure 7.11. The signal from the 2.5 cm (1 in.) radius notch is maximized and is set at the appropriate graticule on the screen display that represents 2.5 cm (1 in.) of sound path (signal A in Figure 7.12). The transducer is then aimed at the 10 cm (4 in.) radius at the end of the IIW block and that signal is set over the graticule representing 10 cm (4 in.) of sound path (signal B in Figure 7.12). By using the range and delay controls as described previously, the two signals are adjusted so that they both align at the proper locations on the screen. For a 12.7 cm (5 in.) screen, the signal from the notch is set a position A over the second major graticule, and the signal from the end radius is set at position B over the eighth major graticule.

Once the screen width is selected and set, the transducer should be placed in position C as shown in Figure 7.11, and the signal from the 0.15 cm (0.06 in.) side-drilled hole maximized. The amplitude of that signal should be set to 80% FSH (or as required by the

(a)

(b)

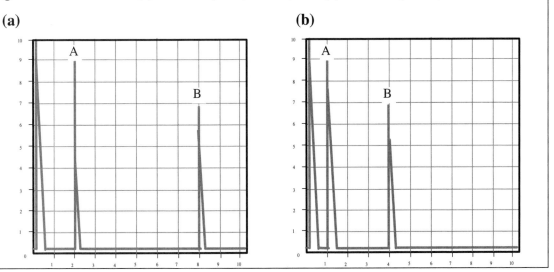

governing code or specification) and that gain setting is recorded as the reference level for the tests performed using this calibration.

With this type of calibration, as opposed to that with a DAC curve, the acceptance and rejection criteria are based on variations in signal amplitude related to sound path. Scanning is done at higher gain settings, as described in the governing code or specification. When an indication is seen, the signal is maximized and the amplitude is set to 80% FSH or whatever FSH percentage was used for calibration. This gain setting is called the *defect level*. The sound path (SP) to the maximized indication is then read from the screen. With these three values, the defect rating can be determined. The defect rating is calculated using the: A–B–C=D, where *A* is the defect level in decibels; *B* is the reference level in decibels; *C* is the attenuation factor; and *D* is the defect rating. The attenuation factor (*C*), is twice the sound path to the indication minus 2.5 cm (1 in.), or $(SP-1)^2$. Here is an example of how this formula is used (in inches).

Assume an indication was found at a sound path of 3 in. The reference level *B* was 40 dB at 80% FSH, and the indication amplitude, when set to 80% FSH required a gain setting of 46 dB (defect level *A*).

Based on this data, *A* would be 46, *B* would be 40, and the attenuation factor *C* would be (3–1) × 2, or 4. Plugging these values into the A–B–C=D formula, we get 46–40–4=2. Therefore, the defect level for this indication would be 2.

The defect rating by itself is just a number (without units); to determine whether or not the indication is rejectable, the governing code or specification has to give ranges of values for rejection. A typical set of ranges might be as follows:

If *D* (defect rating) is less than +5, the indication is rejectable regardless of length. If *D* is from +6 through +9, the indication might be rejectable if the length is greater than 1.9 cm (0.75 in.). If *D* is from +10 through +12, the indication might be rejectable if the length is greater than 5 cm (2 in.). If *D* is greater than +12, the indication might be acceptable regardless of length.

The above ranges are only examples of how a code or specification might define defect ratings. For actual values, the governing code or specification should be consulted.

Distance Sensitivity Calibration Block

A third commonly used calibration block is the distance sensitivity calibration (DSC) block. This block has two radii, 2.5 cm (1 in.) and 7.6 cm (3 in.), as shown in Figure 7.13. The focal point of each radius is at the point where the scribed line on the side of the block hits the scanning surface as shown. To calibrate with this block, the appropriate screen width is selected then the transducer is placed on the flat scanning surface as shown. Several signals will be seen on the screen: from the 2.5 cm (1 in.) radius, from the 7.6 cm (3 in.) radius and from the notch in the 7.6 cm (3 in.) radius.

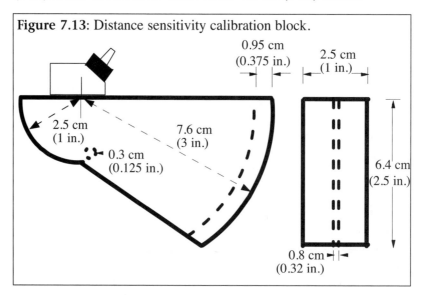

Figure 7.13: Distance sensitivity calibration block.

For a 12.7 cm (5 in.) screen, the signal from the 2.5 cm (1 in.) radius (*A* in Figure 7.14) is maximized and set over the second major graticule, or at a sound path of 2.5 cm (1 in.). The signal coming from the 7.6 cm (3 in.) radius (*B*) is then set over the tenth major graticule (12.7 cm [5 in.] sound path) and the range and delay controls are used to adjust the locations of these signals as described previously. (Note: The signal from the notch will appear just before [to the left of] the signal from the 7.6 cm [3 in.] radius. For now that signal will be ignored.) The transducer is then aimed at the 7.6 cm (3 in.) radius, and if the screen was properly set initially, that signal (*B*) will come up at the sixth major graticule, or at 7.6 cm (3 in.) of sound path. When this occurs, it verifies that the screen width has been accurately set.

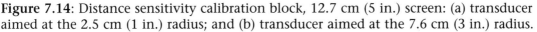

Figure 7.14: Distance sensitivity calibration block, 12.7 cm (5 in.) screen: (a) transducer aimed at the 2.5 cm (1 in.) radius; and (b) transducer aimed at the 7.6 cm (3 in.) radius.

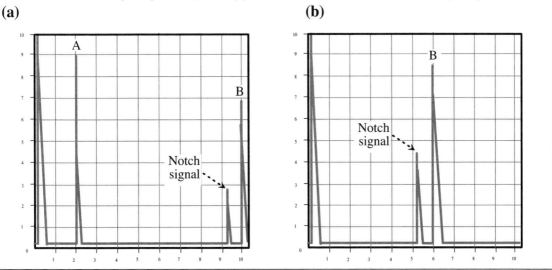

To set up a 25.4 cm (10 in.) screen, the same process is used but with the transducer aimed at the 2.5 cm (1 in.) radius, that signal (*A*) is set over the first major graticule, the first return signal from the 7.6 cm (3 in.) radius (*B*) is set at the fifth major graticule and the second signal from the 7.6 cm (3 in.) radius (*C*) is set at the ninth major graticule. This is shown in the left screen presentation in Figure 7.15. The transducer is then aimed at the 7.6 cm (3 in.) radius and the first signal (*B*) is set over the third major graticule and the second signal (*C*) is set over the seventh major graticule (right screen, Figure 7.15). Signal *A*, from the 2.5 cm (1 in.) radius, does not show on this screen. When the display is adjusted so that these signals all show in the proper location, the 25.4 cm (10 in.) screen width is set. The notch signals will appear just to the left of the radius signals at the seventh and ninth graticules, as shown.

Figure 7.15: Distance sensitivity calibration block, 25.4 cm (10 in.) screen: (a) transducer aimed at the 2.5 cm (1 in.) radius; and (b) transducer aimed at the 7.6 cm (3 in.) radius.

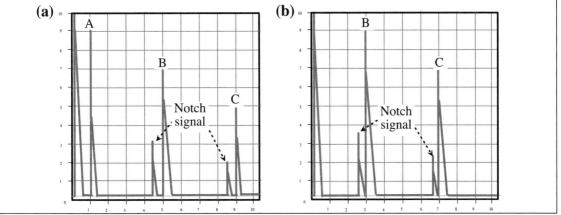

To set the reference level for either screen width, the transducer is aimed at the 7.6 cm (3 in.) radius and the gain control is used to set the signal amplitude from the 3/32 in. (0.23 cm [0.09 in.]) notch to 80% FSH (or as required by the governing code or specification). On the 25.4 cm (10 in.) screen, the first notch signal, just before the third major graticule, is used. As with the IIW block calibration, this calibration uses the A–B–C=D formula and the requirements described previously should be followed.

One question often asked about DSC block calibration is, "Since the larger radius is 7.6 cm (3 in.), why do multiple signals show up at 10.2 cm (4 in.) intervals?" This is due to the nature of reflection and refraction.

When the sound beam hits a material interface at an angle (such as between the wedge and the material being tested), the majority of the sound beam is reflected, with only a small percentage of the sound being sent (refracted) into the second material. The remaining sound reflects back from the interface and ricochets around until it attenuates to zero.

In the DSC block shown in Figure 7.16, the initial sound beam follows arrow A, striking the 2.5 cm (1 in.) radius and returning to the transducer. However, most of the returning sound is reflected down arrow B, striking the 7.6 cm (3 in.) radius and returning back to the scanning surface. That sound beam, which does not hit the scanning surface in the proper orientation to enter the transducer, reflects from the scanning surface down to the 2.5 cm (1 in.) radius as shown by arrow C, then returns to the transducer where it is seen. Because this second trip went to both the 7.6 cm (3 in.) and 2.5 cm (1 in.) radii, the total distance traveled was 10.2 cm (4 in.), which is why the interval between signals is 10.2 cm (4 in.) on the screen display.

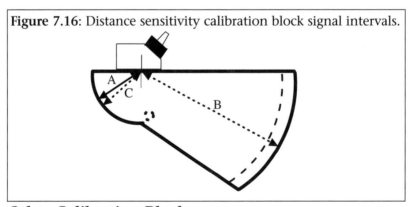

Figure 7.16: Distance sensitivity calibration block signal intervals.

Other Calibration Blocks

There are many other types of calibration blocks available, but most can be used in a similar manner as has been discussed here. Additional information on other calibration blocks can be found in the ASTM International (ASTM) *Book of Standards* Volume 03.03 and in Section V of the American Society of Mechanical Engineers *ASME Boiler & Pressure Vessel Code*.

Chapter 8

Evaluation of Base Material Product Forms

INTRODUCTION

This chapter focuses on various types of materials processing, fabrication and product technology and how they relate to ultrasonic testing. The discussion will focus on ingot pouring and continuous casting followed by the subsequent processes for rolling plate, sheet, bar, rod, pipe and tubular products; forgings, castings, composite structures and weldments; and the discontinuities that might be found in these types of materials and products.

The traditional steel making process starts with iron ore being melted down in blast furnaces to produce molten iron. This iron, often along with scrap steel, is then heated in other furnaces along with lime and various fluxes to create carbon steel. There are alternate processes that do not use molten iron but start with scrap steel and/or other solid feed stocks. The mix resulting from either process is called a *heat* and, in some cases, additional alloying elements such as silicon, nickel, chromium and molybdenum are added to the heat to create specific alloy steels. When the heat is fully mixed and the impurities have been removed (via slag), the furnace is emptied into large fire-brick lined ladles which can be used to fill (cast) ingot molds or are sent to a continuous casting (referred to as *concast*) process.

INGOTS

Ingot molds are large rectangular tapered forms placed on a nonflammable surface, as shown in Figure 8.1. After filling, the molten steel is allowed to cool and solidify into a granular solid. Once the steel has solidified, the molds are removed and the ingots are placed in soaking pits for heating, which equalizes the temperature throughout the ingot. After this process the reheated ingots, are sent to large primary rolling mills to be formed into slabs or billets.

Because the ingots cool from the outside surface inward and the cooling steel contracts, the upper center portion of the ingot often shrinks inward and down into the ingot, causing shrinkage cracks, slag and entrapped gasses. When the gasses are trapped in elongated stringers as they try to come to the surface of the ingot they are called *pipe*, which can extend downward near the center of the ingot.

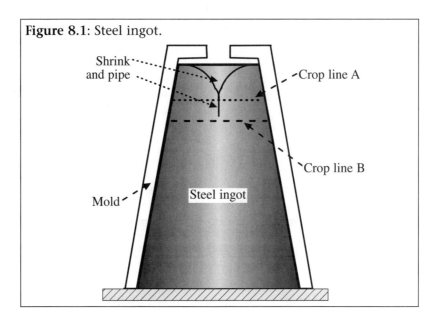

Figure 8.1: Steel ingot.

Shrink and pipe

Crop line A

Crop line B

Mold

Steel ingot

After cooling, the top section of the ingots are cut off, or *cropped*, to remove any shrinkage defects that may have formed during the cooling process. If an ingot is properly cropped, as shown by crop line *B* in Figure 8.1, all of the defective area is removed. If the ingot is cropped too high (crop line *A*), the ingot may still retain some of these defects, a condition that will affect future forming processes.

CONTINUOUS CASTING

Continuous casting is the process in which the ladle of molten steel placed above the casting machine and the steel is poured into an insulated distribution tank called a *tundish*, which in turn feeds the steel into a water-cooled rectangular mold to form a 20 to 30.5 cm (8 to 12 in.) thick slab of steel of a width determined by the size of the casting machine. A representation of the side view of a typical continuous caster is shown in Figure 8.2. Many continuous casters use a turret system that permits ladles to continuously feed the tundish and the casting process can be maintained as long as molten steel can be fed into the tundish, which is why the process is called *continuous casting*.

To initiate this process, a dummy bar is inserted into the base of the mold to act as a floor for the molten steel. As the mold is filled and the outer surfaces of the steel solidify, the dummy bar is slowly pulled down through the curved series of rollers as shown. When the dummy bar passes through the final set of rollers it is removed, leaving a continuous length of new steel extending from the mold to the cutting area beyond the last set of rollers. During the entire casting process, the steel is sprayed with water to control the

Figure 8.2: Continuous caster.

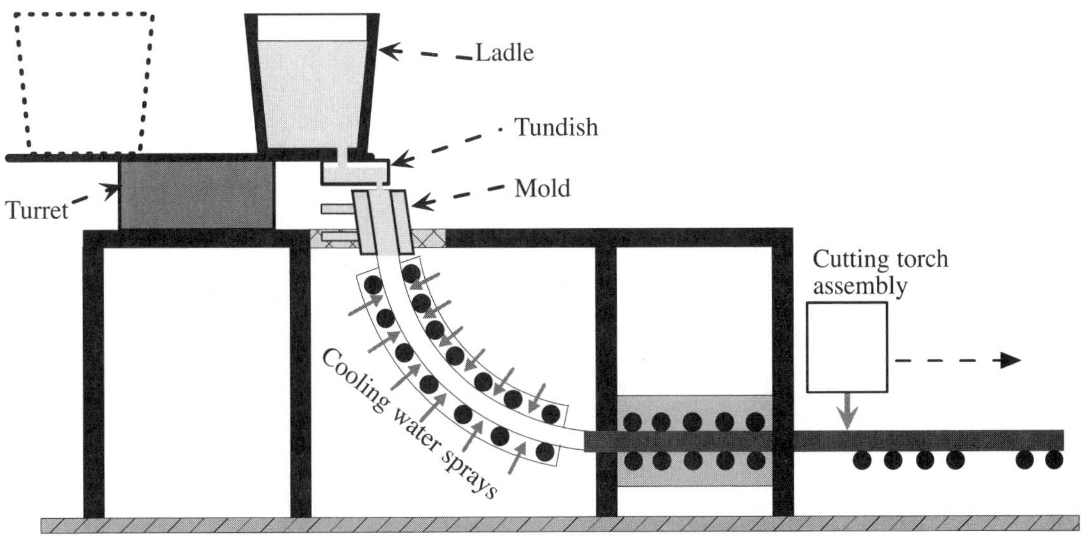

solidification process. Like ingots, the solidification process occurs from the outside inward, so the steel starting down the caster has a solid outer shell with a molten core. As the process continues, the steel solidifies completely and is rolled to the desired thickness as it passes through the final set of rollers. Once the steel exits the final rolls, a cutting torch system clamps to the new slab cutting it to the desired length.

Inherent discontinuities in the ingot casting and continuous casting processes are similar to those of other castings and include segregation, nonmetallic inclusions, shrinkage voids, cracks and pipe.

Segregation occurs when individual elements are either not fully mixed in the heat or separate during the cooling process. Segregated elements do not have the same sound velocity as the parent metal, but unless the areas of segregation are relatively large they cannot be easily seen ultrasonically. Nonmetallic inclusions, such as slag and other contaminants, are generally larger in size than segregations and can be more easily seen using ultrasonic testing.

Shrinkage voids and cracks are both good reflectors of sound and can be seen ultrasonically much more readily than segregation due to the sharp edges of the resulting voids and the large change in sound velocity between the void and the metal. Because the entrapped gas tends to form rounded tubes with smoother sides, pipe does not result in as sharp a reflector as shrinkage and shrink cracks. But because of the change in sound velocity between the gas and the metal, they too can be easily found ultrasonically.

Slabs and Billets

Because of their size, slabs and billets must be processed to reduce them to a manageable thickness. This is done in hot-rolling mills where the heated slab or billet is repeatedly passed through correspondingly tighter rolls. As the slab or billet is rolled it increases in length, resulting in a longer, thinner shape. During this process the metal grains in the steel are elongated in the direction of rolling, as are most discontinuities. Depending on the intended use of the steel, the product may be cut to length between rolling passes to make handling more manageable.

Plate and Sheet

The rolling process permits slabs and billets to be reduced in thickness into plates, and if the process is continued the plate can be rolled into sheets. Since the thinning process continually elongates the product form, rolling sheet steel results in a very long product. To reduce the physical size of the forming area and to make handling easier, the sheet is often formed into a coil. These coils can then be transported, stored for additional forming processes, or sent back through the same rolls set at closer tolerances to further reduce the thickness of the sheet. During the rolling operation several types of process discontinuities can occur, as shown in Figure 8.3.

One such discontinuity is a rolling, or surface, lap which is shown in Figure 8.3a. This occurs when some of the metal humps up in front of one of the rolls (1) then is folded back over the unrolled sheet and pulled through the rolls. This results in an elongated sliver of steel that has been pressed back into the surface of the plate (2). The lap may be visible on close inspection, but may also be smeared closed, making it invisible to the naked eye. During straight beam ultrasonic testing, a lap on the scanning surface side may result in a loss of backwall signal when the transducer passes over it, or may result in a very slight shift in the backwall signal if the lap is on the opposite side of the part from the transducer. If a lap is suspected, magnetic particle testing should also be performed to determine if a lap is present.

Laminations can occur when any of the inherent discontinuities found in ingots, slabs or billets make it into the rolling process. Because the rolling operation compresses the thickness and elongates the material, all such discontinuities are also flattened out and lengthened considerably. Laminations resulting from centerline pipe or shrink remaining after the primary forming process will generally be located close to the center of the thickness of the rolled material, as shown in Figure 8.3b.

Laminations resulting from segregation (Figure 8.3c 1 and 2), or nonmetallic inclusions (Figure 8.3c 3 and 4) may be at any depth in the rolled product. Most laminations can be detected using straight

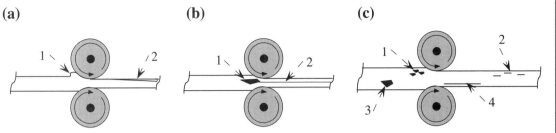

Figure 8.3: Rolling discontinuities: (a) rolling lap; (b) centerline delamination; and (c) segregation and inclusion laminations.

(a)   **(b)**   **(c)**

beam ultrasonic testing, but it should be remembered that all laminations are not continuous across their length or width and may result in intermittent screen signals and/or a loss of backwall signal amplitude (Figure 8.4). On thinner sections, a delay-line transducer may be needed so that the near field effects are contained in the delay line and are not introduced into the test.

Seams are elongated surface discontinuities of varying depth that usually run parallel to the steel rolling direction. They may often be lengthy, are occasionally fissures along the grain and may sometimes be very tight. Being through-thickness in orientation and depending on the depth, seams may be detected using angle beam testing. If extremely shallow, magnetic particle testing is the preferred method, followed by ultrasonic testing to determine depth.

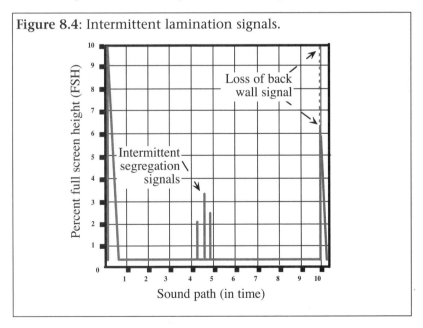

Figure 8.4: Intermittent lamination signals.

BAR AND ROD

The most commonly used process for producing solid round stock (bar and rod) is the rolling process, which is much like the rolling process described for plate and sheet steels. However, since a round product is desired, the rolls in a bar or rod mill have concave contact surfaces (like shallow pulley wheels) rather than flat surfaces. Starting as a heated round ingot or pre-rolled billet, the product moves through a series of consecutively smaller diameter paired rollers that reduce the diameter of the steel while increasing the length. Near the end of the process, some of the rolls may be 90° out from the previous set so that roundness is maintained. As with the sheet rolling process, laps, seams and laminations are the typical inherent discontinuities that are found in these products.

The extrusion process also starts with either a round ingot or a pre-rolled billet that has been heated to an appropriate temperature. The piece is then placed in an extruder similar to the representation shown in Figure 8.5. The ram forces the heated steel through a die the size of the rod or bar that is desired. As the ram advances, the metal is extruded out of the hole in the die plate, creating a rod or bar. Like the rolling process, any discontinuities in the billet will be elongated and compressed during this process. In a similar process, a hot rolled bar or rod can be pulled or drawn through the dies instead of being pushed through. The drawing process is used principally in the manufacture of wire.

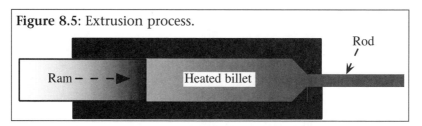

Figure 8.5: Extrusion process.

As with plate and sheet, extruded bar and rod can also have elongated discontinuities such as laminations from nonmetallic inclusions and segregation, and these can also be found ultrasonically. The ultrasonic testing of lengths of round stock is often done using the immersion technique, which involves immersing the test object in de-aerated water treated with anti-corrosion chemicals. Smaller diameter round stock can be passed it through a water box, as shown in Figure 8.6. The rod is pushed through flexible gaskets on either side of a water-filled box, which has one or more search units extending down into the water. The drive rolls spin the rod and drives it through the box at a controlled speed, allowing the search units to interrogate the rod as it passes through the box, using the water in the box to couple the sound beam to the test object. Depending on the number and orientation of search units used, the test object can be tested directly through

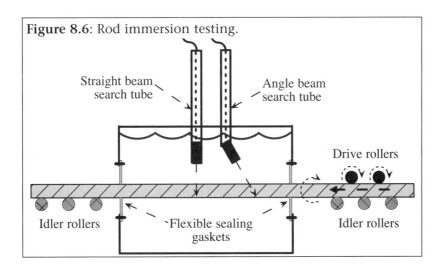

Figure 8.6: Rod immersion testing.

Straight beam search tube

Angle beam search tube

Drive rollers

Idler rollers

Flexible sealing gaskets

Idler rollers

thickness (down the radius), at angles up and down the axis of the test object and at angles around the circumference of the test object in one pass through the box.

For larger diameter round stock, a full immersion tank is used. This setup is similar to the water box, but the entire test object is submersed at one time. The round stock is rotated on fixed (non-moveable) rollers and the ultrasonic machines and search tubes are mounted on a moving assembly called a *bridge*. The bridge can be set to travel at various speeds down the length of the test object and as described above, multiple scans can be performed at one time.

For short pieces of round stock, it may be necessary to perform the test using the contact method. Because the scanning surface is curved, care must be taken to ensure that the transducer is properly coupled to the test object. This can be done by using a contoured wedge that has been curved to match the circumference of the test object, as shown in Figure 8.7. Commercially produced contoured wedges can generally be purchased for standard diameters and can be ordered for any size round stock if time is not a constraint. If necessary, Plexiglas can be cut to the approximate shape then sanded to the exact shape by placing the sandpaper on a piece the same diameter as needed and sanding the wedge until it matches the circumference. One note of caution: When using contoured wedges, calibration can be difficult because a calibration block matching the test object must be used so the technician knows where the sound beam is going.

Hydrogen flakes are fine, circular shaped cracks located near the center of heavy steel forgings, billets and bars that run longitudinally in the steel, as shown in Figure 8.8. Generally found in higher carbon and alloy steels, these flakes result when the cooling process occurs before the dissolved hydrogen can dissipate out of the steel. Straight beam ultrasonic testing is the best method for detecting hydrogen flakes. If there is doubt about the type and location of this discontinuity, the end of the piece may be cut and magnetic particle testing can be done of the cross-section to verify the presence of the flakes.

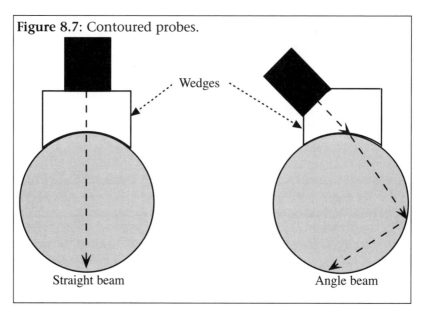

Figure 8.7: Contoured probes.

Wedges

Straight beam

Angle beam

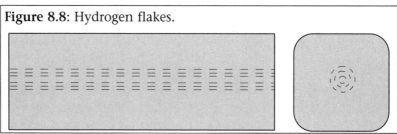

Figure 8.8: Hydrogen flakes.

PIPE AND TUBULAR PRODUCTS

Pipe and tube can be manufactured as seamless or welded product. Seamless pipe and tube in the 15 to 41 cm (6 to 16 in.) diameter range are generally manufactured in a plug mill. In this process, a billet is heated and pierced then a passed through a rotary elongator to form a short, thick-walled hollow tube called a *bloom*. A plug matching the inside diameter of the finished product is placed in the bloom which is then passed through rolls that reduce the thickness, elongating the material as it reduces the thickness. Later rolling processes even out the wall thickness and bring the pipe down to the final thickness.

For seamless product in the 2.5 to 15 cm (1 to 6 in.) range, a mandrel mill is usually used. In this process, an ingot or billet is heated and pierced, then a mandrel is placed in the hole and the assembly is run through a rolling, or mandrel, mill. This differs from a plug mill in that the process is continuous, running between multiple pairs of curved rollers set 90° apart to elongate the material and reduce the wall thickness. The product is then reheated and rolled to final diameter.

The extrusion process is used for small diameter tubes. The round stock is cut to length, heated, sized and descaled, then extruded through a steel die. The material is then run through a reducing mill to obtain the final dimensions and surface finish.

In addition to the inherent discontinuities described previously (laps, voids, laminations and seams), internal tears occasionally occur during the forming process. These crack-like discontinuities will generally be oriented around the inner diameter surface of the pipe or tube and can be found ultrasonically. Typical straight and angle-beam tests are shown in Figure 8.9. Thinning of the pipe wall can also be found using a straight beam thickness test. For thinner walled product, encircling eddy current testing coils are often used instead of ultrasonic testing for discontinuity detection.

Figure 8.9: Contact pipe inspection.

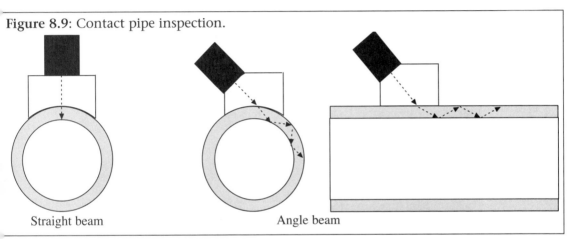

Straight beam   Angle beam

Welded pipe is manufactured by feeding sheet or plate of the proper thickness (called *skelp*) into forming rolls or forms to create a round tube then the edges of the tube are welded, creating a longitudinal or spiral weld seam down the length of the pipe. Weld types will vary depending on the diameter, wall thickness, the manufacturing process and the intended use of the finished product. More common pipe welding processes are electric resistance welding (ERW), including high frequency welding (HFW), and submerged arc welding (SAW). Where submerged arc welding is performed on both the inner diameter and outer diameter of the pipe, the process is called *double submerged arc welding* (DSAW).

Electric resistance and high frequency welds produce a very narrow weld seam, with the most common type of discontinuity being lack of fusion. Hook cracks may occur near the weld line if nonmetallic inclusions are present at the tube edges when the weld is made. Since filler metal and flux is not used in these processes, slag inclusions will not be seen in electric resistance and high frequency welds. Ultrasonic testing of this pipe involves multiple transducers on an automated system testing from both sides of the weld to ensure full weld coverage. Submerged arc welding and double submerged arc welding discontinuities are typical of other electric arc welding processes and will be discussed in the welding section of this chapter.

FORGING

The forging process uses high pressure compressive force to cause plastic deformation of metal into a desired shape. Depending on the size, shape, material type and complexity of the finished test object, the test object may be heated to well above the recrystallization temperature in a range below that temperature or at room temperature. Pressure may be applied by a press, rollers or by repetitive blows of a hammer, depending on the type of forging being done. The basic forging principle is shown in Figure 8.10. Note the grain flow in the test object (arrows in the right figure) as the metal is compressed to fill the die. As with the other forming processes, inherent discontinuities will be stretched and flattened in the direction in which the metal moves.

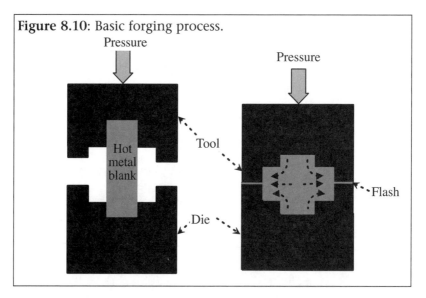

Figure 8.10: Basic forging process.

In addition to the distortion of inherent discontinuities, processing discontinuities such as forging bursts and hot tears can also occur in the forging process. Forging bursts occur when the metal being worked cannot withstand the tensile stress that occurs during the forging process. Bursts vary in size, may be open cavities or like tight cracks and may be oriented longitudinally or transversely, as shown at the left in Figure 8.11. Cracking may occur when there is differential cooling at changes in thickness, as shown at the right in Figure 8.11. Both types of discontinuities can be found ultrasonically using either straight or angle beam testing, or a combination of both.

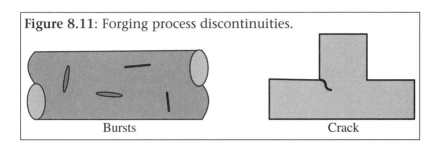

Figure 8.11: Forging process discontinuities.

Bursts

Crack

CASTINGS

The casting process involves melting the metal and pouring or injecting the molten material into a mold of the desired shape. Ingot casting, as discussed earlier, is one of the simpler forms of casting, but molds can be designed for extremely complex shapes and may vary in size from finger-sized objects up to shapes the size of a house.

A simplified representation of the sand casting process is shown in Figure 8.12. The mold is formed around a pattern in the desired shape, then molten metal is poured into the pouring cup. The metal flows through the vertical sprue into the gating system, filling the mold cavity. The riser holds additional metal so that when the metal contracts as it cools there is sufficient metal to fill the mold, preventing shrinkage cavities (described below).

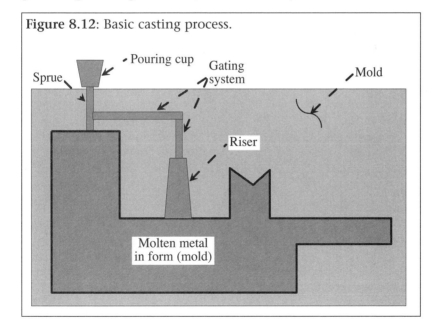

Figure 8.12: Basic casting process.

Pouring cup

Gating system

Mold

Sprue

Riser

Molten metal in form (mold)

Typical discontinuities found in castings are shown by number in Figure 8.13 and are defined by number as follows.

1. Porosity is usually caused by the release of dissolved gasses as the molten metal cools, creating bubbles or pores. Pores are generally small diameter with smooth surfaces. Multiple pores in one area are called *cluster porosity*, and if the porosity is moving as the metal cools, the porosity may form an elongated void commonly called *piping* (or *worm-hole*) porosity, as shown.

2. Gas holes are created in the same manner as porosity but are larger in diameter and generally tend to be isolated or limited in the number found in any one area.

3. Inclusions are areas where nonmetallic materials such as slag or sand are trapped in the material as the metal cools.

4. Hot tears are crack-like tears that occur when the material starts to contract during the initial cooling phase, just below the solidification temperature. If the hardening material is restrained by the mold at that point, the material may tear, usually at changes in section where a stress-riser already exists.

5. Cracks are irregularly shaped, linear defects (fractures) that can be caused when internal stresses exceed the strength of the material. In the casting process, stress cracks can occur due to contraction, residual stress, shock or due to inservice stresses.

6. Shrinkage cavities occur when the liquid metal contracts and solidifies during cooling. If there is not enough molten metal to offset the resulting contraction, the metal may pull apart, creaking a void or cavity in the solidified material. These typically occur where additional molten metal cannot be fed in quickly enough to offset the contraction, or where there are variations in section thickness.

7. Air pockets occur when the air in the unfilled mold cannot escape as the molten metal is added. These generally are found near the top surface of the object just beneath the surface.

8. Cold shuts are areas where part of the filler material solidifies before mold cavity is completely filled. As additional molten material reaches the already cooled section of metal it may not fuse together, forming a tight line of disbond between the two segments of metal. In the welding processes, this would be considered lack of fusion.

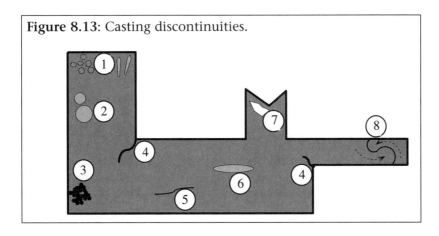

Figure 8.13: Casting discontinuities.

Because of the nature of the casting and cooling process, there is a tendency for the material to have larger grain sizes than materials formed in other processes. If the finished product is not subjected to additional heat treatment processes to refine (reduce) the grain size, this can present a problem when ultrasonic testing is done. In coarser materials such as cast iron, the grain size may be sufficiently large and coarse to cause the sound beam to reflect from the grains, causing the sound beam to scatter inside the test object with a resultant loss of returned sound. In cases like this, ultrasonic testing technicians might believe that they are performing a full test, when in fact the sound is not fully penetrating the test object. This is one of the reasons why the calibration block material is required to be as close a metallurgical match (ultrasonically equivalent) to the test object possible.

COMPOSITES (BONDED STRUCTURES)

Composites are formed by joining two or more layers (plies) of materials with different physical or chemical properties into one bonded assembly, as shown in Figure 8.14. Composites are commonly used in applications that require high strength, lightweight materials. By combining different materials into a composite sandwich, the advantages of the properties of multiple materials can be incorporated into a single product. Composites are used in an extremely wide range of applications, varying from plywood to the reinforced carbon-carbon (RCC) composites.

The most common discontinuities (see Figure 8.14) found in composites are delaminations, foreign material inclusions and porosity. Delamination, or the separation of plies, can result from shock loading, impact or cyclic stresses. This can also result in fiber pull-out where individual fibers separate from the composite matrix. The inclusion of foreign materials can occur if the composite materials are not kept clean or are mishandled during the material assembly process prior to the fusing of the base materials into one

Figure 8.14: Composites and discontinuities.

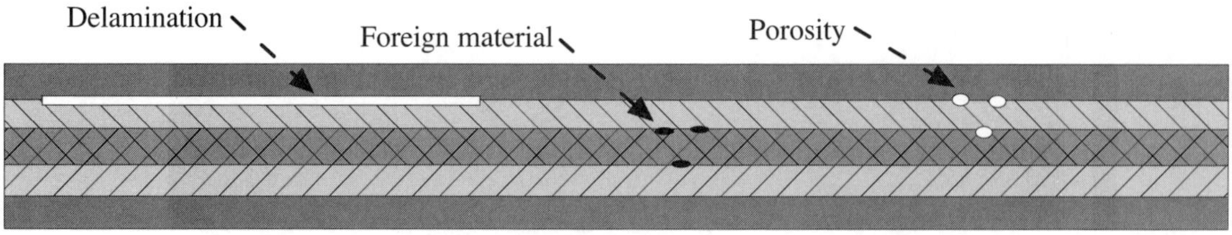

substance. Such inclusions are not only tiny areas of disbond, but can create stress risers that may lead to delamination. Porosity can occur when the base materials outgas during the fusing process and all of the gasses do not escape the composite before it hardens. This can also lead to weak areas that could lead to further failure.

Depending on the materials used to create a composite, ultrasonic testing can be used to test these structures. If the composite is thin, it may be necessary to use a delay line in front of the transducer or switch to an immersion technique so that the near field effects are contained in the delay line or water path and are not introduced into the testing.

WELDS

Welding is the most commonly used metals joining method in industry, and welds are the most common structural item to be ultrasonically tested under shop or field conditions. As a result, it is important that ultrasonic testing technicians have a basic knowledge of the most commonly used welding processes, and that they be familiar with standard welding terminology. Prior to performing ultrasonic testing on a weld, the technician should ask which weld process was used to make the weld(s). Knowing this, and knowing what discontinuities can occur in the various types of weld, can prevent a technician from calling out a discontinuity that couldn't exist in the weld due to the weld process that was used. Miss-calls of this nature tend to lead to a loss of credibility for the technician.

Welding Terminology

Figure 8.15 shows several of the more common weld joint configurations used in industry. Welds *A* through *E* show butt welds, so named because the two pieces of base metal are butted up against each other prior to welding. The edges of the plate(s) are grooved to permit access to the bottom of the weld, which is why butt welds are often called *groove welds*. If the weld is designed to fill the full thickness of the test objects, the weld is called a *full penetration weld*. If the weld is designed to penetrate only part way through the material thickness, as shown in weld *E*, the joint is called a *partial penetration weld*. Partial penetration welds are hard to test

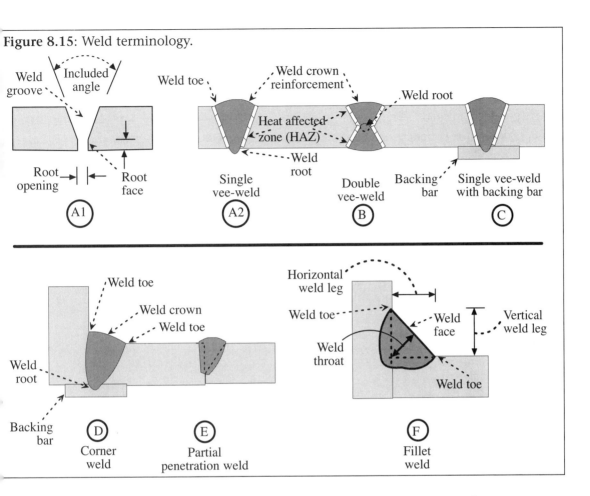

Figure 8.15: Weld terminology.

ultrasonically (if the governing code or specification permits it at all) because the ultrasonic test signal from the gap at the root of a partial penetration weld can mask discontinuities actually in the weld root. If the groove in the base material is all from one side, the weld is designated as a single-vee weld, as shown in welds *A*, *C* and *D*, and the root opening is at the bottom of the weld. If the joint is grooved on both sides, as shown in weld *B*, the weld is called a *double-vee weld* and the root is in the center of the weld thickness. Because the root is the hardest part of a weld to make, many of the weld discontinuities found will tend to be at the root, so it is important for the ultrasonic testing technician to know the location of the root. Knowing the included angle of the original weld groove can aid the ultrasonic testing technician in determining which wedge angle will be best for detecting side-wall fusion discontinuities.

Weld *F* is a fillet weld that is not deposited in a groove, but is placed in a corner formed by the base material. Because the majority of the weld metal is deposited above the base metal and there is an inherent gap at the root of the weld, these welds do not lend themselves well to ultrasonic testing.

Along the edge of every weld is an area in the base metal called the *heat affected zone* (HAZ). The heat affected zone is that area of the base material immediately adjacent to the weld that has been heated to a temperature high enough to affect the mechanical properties or change the microstructure of the metal but below the melting point. Examples of the effects of this heating can be refined grain structure and changes in the hardness, ductility or strength of the steel. The width of the HAZ will vary depending on the amount of heat input into the weld, inter-pass temperatures and cooling rate. Because this area is susceptible to change, most codes and specifications require that an inch or so of the base metal also be included in area of interest for the ultrasonic test.

Welding Processes

In some welding processes, no filler metal is used and the weld is formed by melting the edges of the two pieces of base metal together. These are called *non-consumable processes* since no filler metal is used. When filler metal is added to form the weld by burning off the electrode, it is considered a *consumable process*. All welds involve melting the base metal to a molten state and allowing it to join with other molten metal (or itself) then cooling to form a single piece. In the electric arc welding process, current is passed through the welding electrode to complete a circuit with the base material, resulting in a high temperature electric arc forming between the base metal and electrode.

Because the molten metal is susceptible to contamination during the welding process, the molten metal must be shielded from atmospheric contaminants during welding. To do this, the weld area is shielded from the atmosphere by either supplying shielding gasses released by melting various chemical elements that have been combined together to form a flux, by flooding the weld area with an inert gas (or a combination of gasses) or a combination of both. When flux is used, the shielding gas is given off by the melting flux and the remaining melted solids cool to form a glass-like coating over the weld, called *slag*, which helps reduce the cooling rate of the weld metal. When multiple layers (passes) of weld material are required, this slag must be removed completely between passes to prevent having it re-melted and mixed back into the next layer of weld or trapped between layers, creating slag inclusions.

Figure 8.16 shows examples of this shielding along with the five most commonly used welding processes used in shop fabrication and field erection:

1. Shielded metal arc welding (SMAW).
2. Submerged arc welding (SAW).
3. Gas tungsten arc welding (GTAW).
4. Gas metal arc welding (GMAW).
5. Flux-cored arc welding (FCAW).

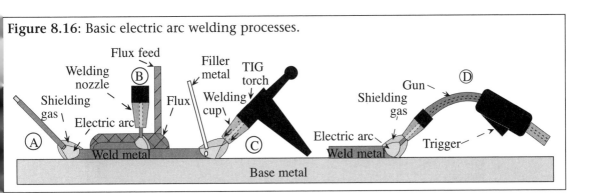

Figure 8.16: Basic electric arc welding processes.

The SMAW process (commonly called *stick welding*) is shown in Figure 8.16a. This process uses a straight piece of welding electrode (rod), coated with a covering of chemical elements to form a flux, as described previously. Electrode length varies based on the diameter of the steel core, but the most commonly used electrode sizes are 35.5 cm (14 in.) in length. Since the electrode holder (stinger) grips the back end of the rod, not all of the rod can be consumed in the weld, with a common stub length being between 5 and 10 cm (2 and 4 in.), with the length varying depending on the accessibility of the weld groove.

To make a stick weld, the rod is placed in an electrode holder and the other end is scratched across the surface were the weld is wanted to create the electric arc. As the rod burns off, a pool of molten metal, or puddle, is formed and the welder continues to feed the electrode into the puddle and move that puddle down the weld groove to create the weld. Due to the brightness of the arc and the presence of very strong ultraviolet radiation, welders are required to protect their eyes and skin from burns.

Figure 8.16b shows the submerged arc welding (SAW) process, where a solid welding wire is fed from a spool down through feed rollers and through a welding nozzle. Granular flux is fed from a flux hopper into the weld groove just ahead of the weld nozzle so that the welding wire makes contact with the base metal beneath a mound of flux. The arc is established under that flux mound, melting the flux immediately around the arc, creating the shielding gasses required to protect the molten weld metal. As with the SMAW process, the melted flux cools to become slag which must be removed between passes. Excess flux that was not melted can be recovered, reconditioned and reused. Because the arc is fully shielded by the flux covering the weld groove, welding technicians are not required to use eye protection if the process is operating properly. This process is usually only used in the flat position because of the need to have the flux stay on the weld. When the proper set-up parameters are used, this automated welding process can produce large amounts of continuous weld. However, if the set-up parameters are incorrect, for example, if the weld nozzle is misaligned with the weld groove, long lengths of bad weld can also be made, usually with the same discontinuity over the length of that weld.

Figure 8.16c shows the gas tungsten arc welding (GTAW) process. This process was formerly called the tungsten inert gas (TIG) process (and still is by some welders), but since other non-inert gasses are now used for shielding this terminology is no longer accurate. The GTAW process was so named because the non-consumable welding electrode is made of tungsten. The shielding gas comes from external gas bottles and flows through tubing to the torch handle and out through the welding cup, beside the electric lead back to the power source. When filler metal is required, it is usually a thin bare wire fed into the weld puddle by hand.

Figure 8.16d shows the set-up for both the gas metal arc welding (GMAW) and the flux-cored arc welding (FCAW) processes. These two processes use similar equipment but have different shielding processes. The GMAW process was formerly called the metal inert gas (MIG) welding process since the original gasses used were inert. Like GTAW, other gasses are now used as shielding and this terminology is inaccurate. (Note: In some countries, this process is called *MIG/MAG*, which denotes metal inert gas/metal active gas welding.)

With GMAW, the shielding gasses are fed to the welding gun (so-called because there is a wire-feed trigger on it) by tube as is done in the GTAW process. However, instead of having a non-consumable electrode like GTAW, wire is fed from an external spool through the gun and out of a nozzle in a manner similar to the SAW process. The wire feed speed is set at the spool controls and the welder starts both the gas and the wire feed by squeezing the trigger on the handle of the gun. When properly set, the shielding gas starts flowing just before the wire starts to feed so that the shielding gasses are in place when the arc ignites.

The flux-cored arc welding (FCAW) process also uses a gun like GMAW, but as the name implies, the filler wire is tubular not solid, containing a central core of fine granular flux. FCAW that is without shielding gas is said to be self-shielding and is designated as FCAW-S. If an external gas is used, the process is designated FCAW-G. With the exception of needing slightly larger wire feed drive rollers and contact tips (the copper tube inside the gun nozzle that conducts the electricity to the wire), the equipment is essentially the same as that used in the GMAW process.

Weld Discontinuities

Prior to performing angle beam tests, a straight beam test of the scanning surface is generally required by most codes and specifications. The purpose of this scan is to determine that the base metal beneath the angle beam transducer does not contain discontinuities, particularly laminations that might interfere with the angle beam testing. If the base metal is laminated, the sound beam may reflect from the lamination rather than the back wall, resulting in the condition shown in Figure 8.17. If this occurs and is not caught prior to testing, the technician will not have any idea where the sound beam is actually going, rendering any interpretation impossible.

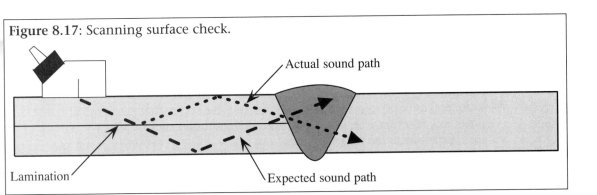

Figure 8.17: Scanning surface check.

Knowing the types of discontinuities that can occur in the various types of welds will help technicians understand what types of discontinuities may be expected in the weld. Table 8.1 shows the various discontinuities that can be found in the previously discussed weld processes, followed by descriptions of the various discontinuity types and how they may appear during ultrasonic testing. These descriptions are general in nature since every discontinuity has its own individual characteristics, but the screen displays shown are typical of the screen presentations that may be seen when these discontinuities are encountered. Actual screen displays will vary based on discontinuity size, orientation and location, and technicians should remember that the interpretation of the ultrasonic testing screen signals is a learned art, not a science. In many cases there may be multiple discontinuity types at the same location, such as a crack running out of a slag inclusion or slag mixed in with porosity, so it is often impossible to state positively what discontinuity is actually being seen, which is why the term *interpretation* is used.

Table 8.1: Welding process discontinuities.

Welding Process	Cracks	Incomplete penetration	Lack of fusion	Porosity	Slag inclusions	Tungsten inclusions	Undercut
Shielded metal arc welding (SMAW)	X	X	X	X	X		X
Submerged arc welding (SAW)	X	X	X	X	X		X
Gas tungsten arc welding (GTAW)	X	X	X	X		X	X
Gas metal arc welding (GMAW)	X	X	X	X			X
Flux-cored arc welding-self shielded (FCAW-S)	X	X	X	X	X		X
Flux-cored arc welding-gas shielded (FCAW-G)	X	X	X	X	X		X

The inability to be able to always identify a discontinuity type is a constant irritation to owners and contractors, but the truth of the matter is that if the size of a discontinuity exceeds the governing acceptance criteria it will have to be removed regardless of the discontinuity type. On the other hand, many codes and specifications state that any crack, lack of fusion or incomplete penetration is rejectable regardless of size, so under those conditions discontinuity identification can be critical, and technicians will only become proficient in this with experience.

Cracks occur when stresses exceed the strength of the material, resulting in a tear or rupture in that material that are usually irregularly shaped with jagged edges that make good ultrasonic reflectors. Cracks generally initiate at a surface and propagate into the material, but if there is an internal discontinuity or stress riser it may create a focal point for those stresses and a crack may start at that point. Figure 8.18 shows how a signal from a crack on the opposite of the plate will walk across the screen of the ultrasonic testing machine.

As the sound beam approaches the crack (*A*), the sound beam is just beginning to hit the crack. Because the sound path from the leading edge of the sound beam is longer than the sound path along the centerline of the beam, the screen signal appears at the far right side of the screen. The signal will move to the left, gaining amplitude until the centerline of the beam hits the corner formed by the crack and the bottom of the plate (*B*). As the sound beam continues past the crack, the signal continues to move to the left, dropping in amplitude until the sound beam clears the crack and the signal drops off the screen.

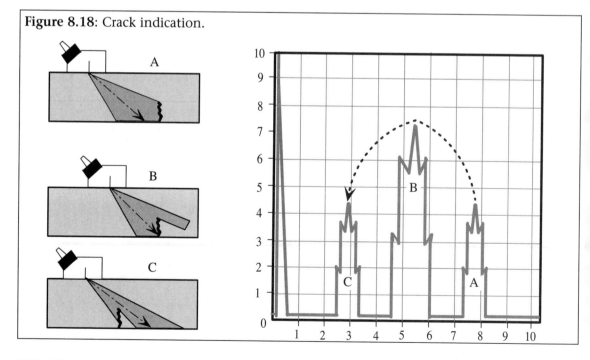

Figure 8.18: Crack indication.

This is typical of a crack signal, but depending on the thickness of the test object or whether the crack is seen in the second leg of the sound beam, this sequence may occur over a much shorter segment of the screen. The depth (height) of the crack will also affect the signal amplitude. Because most cracks have jagged surfaces, the left edge of the signal may be stair-stepped as shown, created a steeple-shaped signal on the screen.

Crater cracks are small shrink cracks that can occur in the weld puddle (crater) at the end of a weld bead that has not been fully filled. They may be a single linear discontinuity or may have multiple cracks forming a star-shaped indication. These discontinuities are often shallow, and being on the top surface of the weld, are hard to detect ultrasonically due to interference from the weld's surface contour. Visual or magnetic particle testing is best for detecting this type of crack.

Incomplete penetration (IP) occurs when the weld metal does not fully penetrate the weld groove root area, leaving all or a portion of the original root face undisturbed, as shown in Figure 8.19. As the transducer is moved toward the single-vee groove weld from the left side, the forward (or upper) portion of the beam cone encounters the root face at transducer position *A* and produces a screen deflection that matches the sound path distance from the beam index point (BIP) of the transducer to the root face along the top edge of the beam cone (signal position *A* on the screen).

In the course of typical scanning, the transducer is moved closer to the weld toward transducer position *B*, and the signal that initiated at screen position *A* grows in amplitude until it maximizes at screen position *B* in response to the increased sound energy in the center of the beam cone, intercepting the corner reflector formed by the discontinuity. (The maximum height of the reflection from this point will typically cause the technician to place a reference mark on the test surface and perform the math function necessary to prove exact position of the reflector).

As the transducer is moved closer to the weld (to transducer position *C*), the signal amplitude and position will decrease toward screen position *C*. This is because the lower portion of the sound beam cone is weaker than the center portion. As the movement of the transducer progresses toward position *C*, the beam cone centerline is moving above the primary reflective surfaces of the discontinuity; thus the lower amplitude of the screen signal position *C*. The lessened sound path of position *C* is a measure of the distance between the BIP and the discontinuity along the lower edge of the sound beam cone.

When approached from the other side of the single-vee weld (transducer position *D*), forward movement of the transducer will be stopped by the weld crown, preventing full coverage of the root area. As shown, only the upper portion of the beam cone will actually contact the flawed area of the root. In such a case, the discontinuity signal will be seen to be rising, but contact with the crown will interfere with further evaluation unless the weld crown is ground flush or a higher angle (70°) transducer is used.

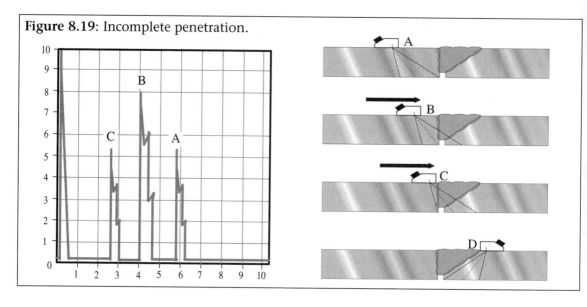

Figure 8.19: Incomplete penetration.

Because incomplete penetration is caused by the original weld groove not being fully melted, the reflecting surfaces of the discontinuity are much smoother than those of a crack. Consequently, the left edge of the screen signal will tend to be more vertical instead of exhibiting the steeple shape often found with cracks.

Lack of fusion is a discontinuity that occurs when the molten weld metal does not fuse in to the base metal or previous weld layer. Sidewall lack of fusion occurs when the weld metal does not fuse in to the side of the weld groove, leaving a smooth, planar discontinuity along the edge of the weld groove, which is shown in the top section of Figure 8.20. When molten weld metal does not tie in to another weld bead, the condition is called *innerbead lack of fusion*, which is shown in the bottom portion of Figure 8.20.

Sidewall lack of fusion is usually best seen ultrasonically in the second leg from the same side of the weld (transducer position *A1*). Because the sound beam is coming up from the bottom surface, it tends to hit the lack of fusion more nearly perpendicular to the flat surface which gives the best reflection. In the first leg (*A2*), the sound is more nearly parallel to the plane of the discontinuity, causing the majority of the sound to flow past or reflect downward from the discontinuity into the test object, away from the transducer. Some sound may return, causing a screen signal to appear, but it may have insufficient amplitude to cause the lack of fusion to be ruled rejectable.

When the weld is scrubbed from the opposite side of the weld in the second leg (*D1*), the sound beam is again more nearly parallel to the plane of the lack of fusion, again with minimal sound return. In the first leg (*D2*), it is possible that the transducer may bump into the weld crown prior to being close enough for the sound beam to hit the discontinuity. However, if the lack of fusion is located lower down in the weld, a very solid signal may be seen since the sound beam would hit the lack of fusion nearly perpendicular to the flat surface (as it did

Figure 8.20: Lack of fusion.

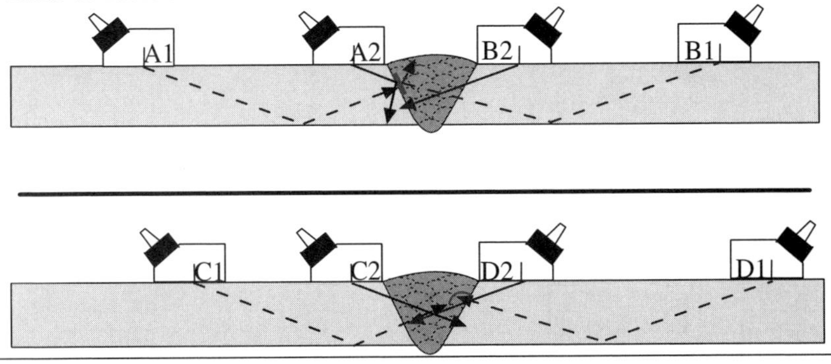

in the second leg from *A1*). If a strong second-leg signal is seen that indicates the probability of sidewall lack of fusion in the upper portion of the weld, the technician may need to have the weld crown ground flush so the weld can be re-tested from the other side in the first leg.

Innerbead lack of fusion can be much harder to locate and identify because it does not lie up flush against the groove sidewall but may be in any orientation between weld beads, is usually non-planar and will only be as smooth as the crown of the previous weld bead. As with sidewall lack of fusion (or any discontinuity, for that matter), if the discontinuity is near the top of the weld it will not be seen in the first leg of the sound beam. This is shown in the bottom section of Figure 8.20.

At transducer location *C1*, the sound beam is nearly parallel to the plane of the discontinuity and the amount of sound reflected back to the transducer will be minimal. A position *C2*, the transducer hits the toe of the weld crown, preventing the sound beam from seeing the discontinuity. At position *D1*, the second leg of the sound beam will hit the discontinuity and the discontinuity can be evaluated. However, if this indication cannot be verified from any other position, it may be necessary to grind the weld crown flush so that the indication can be evaluated in the first leg.

Porosity was defined previously under the castings section of this chapter as small gas pores in the weld metal. Formed when gas is trapped in the weld before it can float to the surface, pores are generally rounded voids with a smooth internal surface. Because of the round, smooth shape, sound will generally hit small pores as a single point contact, as shown in Figure 8.21a-c. At point (*A*), the sound beam is just coming over the pore and the sound on the edge of the beam hits the pore at a slight angle, causing that sound to reflect away from the transducer and it is not seen. As the centerline of the sound beam hits the pore squarely (*B*), sound is reflected back and the indication is seen on the screen, then as the sound beam moves past (*C*), what sound does hit the pore will reflect back behind the transducer and will not be seen. Because this occurs at a single point on a small pore, the signal is usually a single, discrete vertical line the pops up at one point on the screen then drops off without moving sideways.

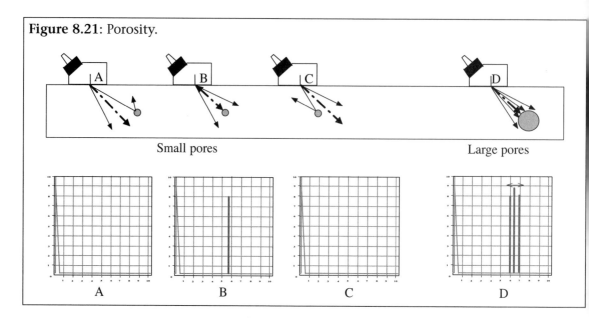

Figure 8.21: Porosity.

Small pores   Large pores

A   B   C   D

Larger gas pores will result in a slightly different screen display. If the pore is sufficiently large, the surface curvature, being flatter, will reflect more sound. The signal will peak as with a small pore, but may also move to the left slightly as the sound beam passes over it (*D*). When maximizing the signal from a large pore, the single signal will walk back and forth sideways over a small portion of the screen with the maximum amplitude being at the center of that space.

Cluster porosity is just that, a group or cluster of pores near each other in the weld, as shown in Figure 8.22. Each pore is a discrete round discontinuity that reflects sound like a single pore. However, since there are multiple discontinuities, the screen will show multiple single spikes as the sound beam passes over the cluster. If the pores are small, each signal will pop up and disappear at the same point on the screen, with adjacent signals increasing or decreasing in amplitude at the same time. The lateral spacing on the signals on the screen will vary based on the individual distance from each pore to the transducer.

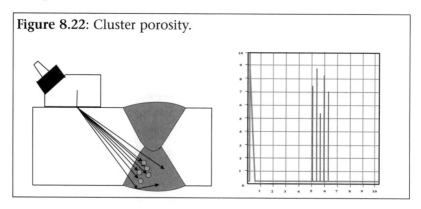

Figure 8.22: Cluster porosity.

Slag inclusions are seen in two forms: solid slag that is left from a previous weld pass, or molten slag that is trapped when the weld metal solidifies before the slag can float to the surface of the weld. These slag types are shown in the weld cross-section in Figure 8.23.

Slag that has been left on a previous weld pass (*A*) usually occurs when the welder has not completely cleaned the earlier weld pass and then welds over that slag without re-melting it, preventing it from floating up through the molten weld puddle. This type of slag may have semi-sharp edges and may be in fairly long stringers parallel to the weld length. Slag that is trapped in the cooling weld metal (*B*) tends to be more rounded and is often oblong or oval in shape. This type of slag is generally smooth sided (similar to a pore) but may contain gas as well as solids.

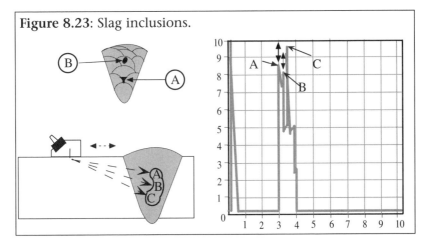

Figure 8.23: Slag inclusions.

Slag signals on the screen often show up as a cluster of side-by-side screen signals with individual signal amplitudes that vary in height as the sound beam passes over the slag. The signals from the peanut-shaped piece of slag shown at the bottom left of Figure 8.23 will give the signals shown on the screen presentation. (The slag shown has been enlarged to illustrate a typical peanut-shaped contour.) Point *A*, at the top of the slag, is closer to the transducer and has a convex surface facing the sound beam so it tends to give a fairly sharp signal. The sound hitting point *B* hits a concave surface that is just slightly farther from the transducer, and that signal tends to be focused by the curvature of the slag surface with the focal point being closer than the transducer, so less sound returns to the transducer. Being slightly lower in the weld than *A*, point *B* is farther from the transducer so that signal falls immediately to the right of the *A* signal on the screen. Point *C*, at the bottom of the slag, is again convex, like *A*, so it too can give a good sound return resulting in a higher amplitude than *B*. However, it is farther from the transducer than *B*, so that signal falls just to the right of the *B* signal on the screen.

As the transducer is moved forward and starts to hit the slag inclusion, the signal amplitude will increase as the center of the sound beam crosses each point on the slag. Because the sound path is shortening as the transducer approaches, the cluster of signals will walk across the screen to the left until the sound beam clears the slag. As this happens, the signal height for each reflector will drop off until they drop off the screen.

Tungsten inclusions are metallic inclusions that occur when the tip of the tungsten electrode melts off and drops into the weld puddle. These are usually more or less round and can give a screen signal similar to that of a gas pore, though the metal-to-metal interface does not give near as good a reflection as does a pore.

Undercut is a condition that usually occurs when the welding amperage is too high, resulting in the top of the groove at the toe of the weld being burned away, leaving a depression along the edge of the weld. This condition can usually be seen visually, and when ultrasonic testing is performed may result in a signal from the toe of the weld. Since the undercut can mask other discontinuities at that location, if a toe signal is seen where undercut is present it should be removed by grinding to confirm that the undercut caused the screen signal.

False Indications

Verification of weld soundness and the identification of discontinuities (if present) is the primary purpose of performing ultrasonic testing. The second most important goal is to leave good weld in place, i.e., not rejecting good welds due to indications that may be caused by conditions other than discontinuities. Removing and replacing good welds is an unnecessary expense for the fabricator, and making such calls ruins the credibility of the technician. Three common conditions that create false calls will be discussed here: misinterpretation of backing bar signals, mode conversion and the presence of external reflectors.

Backing bars are commonly used in butt welds on structural steel. The purpose of the bar is to provide a surface under the weld groove for the welder to use to lay the first bead (root pass) of the weld. A properly welded backed butt joint will result in full penetration between the sidewalls of the weld and the backing bar. As a result, sound will enter the backing bar through this weld junction, and due to the geometry may ricochet off the corners of the backing then return to the transducer. Figure 8.24 shows this joint configuration and how the sound beam may reflect back from a corner. The signal from a backing bar reflector, since it is below the bottom edge of the plate, will appear to be in the second leg of the sound beam, with how far it is in the second leg depending on which corner is causing the reflection. Because this signal occurs just into the second leg, this signal may be misidentified as a sidewall discontinuity.

Technicians can check for this condition in three ways. First, the weld should be tested from the opposite side if at all possible. If that

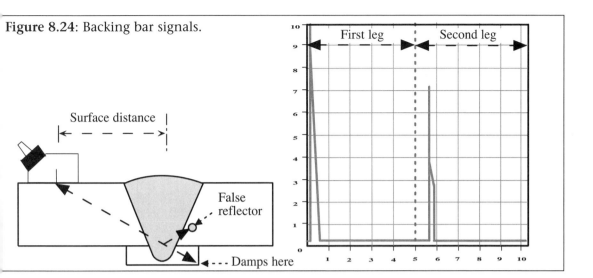

Figure 8.24: Backing bar signals.

is not possible, such as when the weld is a corner weld, other means must be used. If the backing bar is accessible, a technique called *damping* can be used, which involves wetting a finger with couplant then tapping the backing bar corner below and in front of the transducer. If the sound beam is reflecting from that corner, the signal amplitude will drop slightly (usually about 5 to 10% FSH) as the corner is tapped. This occurs because some of the sound will enter the wet finger, causing less sound to reflect back which decreases the signal amplitude. The second method of verification is to compare the sound path to the surface distance (see Figure 8.24). If the signal is from the backing bar, this comparison will show that the surface distance is too short for the sound path and the suspected discontinuity would actually be in the base material on the far side of the weld, not in the weld.

One indicator that suggests this signal is from the backing bar is the height of the screen signal. Because a corner makes a really good reflector, the amplitude of the signal from a backing bar is usually quite high, often exceeding 100% FSH even at reference level. Under most conditions, sidewall discontinuities will not reflect near that amount of sound, so when such a signal is seen, the presence of a backing bar reflector must be considered.

Mode conversion is another phenomenon that can cause false reflectors. Mode conversion occurs when a change in angle causes the shear wave to convert to a longitudinal wave. This can occur in a weld when the sound beam hits a reflector so oriented to cause the wave mode to change. Two typical examples of mode conversion in welds are shown on the left side of Figure 8.25. In the top sketch, the sound beam reflects from the gap between the backing bar, the weld and the base metal. In the bottom left sketch, the sound reflects from the root reinforcement.

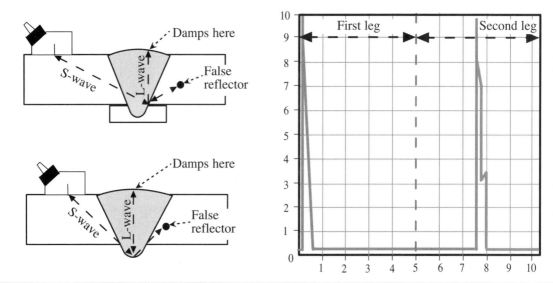

Figure 8.25: Backing bar signals.

In both cases, the change in angle is such that the shear wave sound beam converts to a longitudinal wave, reflects up to the top weld crown then returns to the root, converts back to a shear wave then returns to the transducer.

Since the velocity of a longitudinal wave is approximately twice that of a shear wave, the signal generated by the weld crown appears to be in the second leg of the sound beam at a distance of about half the thickness of the weld. The result is a very strong screen signal that appears near the middle of the second leg. As with backing bar signals, if technicians plot the surface distance and the sound path, they see that this false indication falls outside the weld zone in the base metal on the opposite side of the weld. Additionally, if the damping technique is used on the weld crown, the screen signal amplitude should change appreciably when the surface is tapped.

External attachments can be another cause of false indications. Figure 8.26 shows several examples of this type of false indication that can occur in a typical structural beam-column moment connection with a corner butt weld. In this case, a gusset plate was fillet welded between the column flanges in the shop to carry the load across the gap and the moment connections were made in the field.

At transducer positions *A* and *B*, the sound beam passes through the weld and column flange, hitting the faces of the gusset plate fillet welds and then returns to the transducer. At transducer position *C*, the sound beam has hit the upper corner of the cope hole and returned to the transducer. (Cutting a cope hole out of the web is a common practice to provide space to install a continuous backing bar under the weld.) All three of these indications can be damped at the locations shown by the circled *D*.

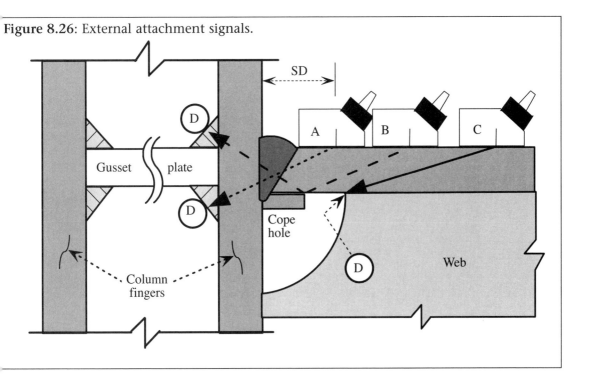

Figure 8.26: External attachment signals.

At positions *A* and *B*, the surface distance from the column face is obviously much too short to have such a second leg signal, and at *C* the surface distance is far too long for a first leg signal to be coming from the weld. When signals such as these occur, technicians must consider that some outside influence is affecting the sound beam, and the simplest means to determine this is to look on the back side of the test object, in this case the column flange. Similar external reflectors can occur in other applications, such as lifting lugs welded to the opposite side on the shell on an above-ground tank, attachments to the inside of pressure vessel, etc. If the opposite side of the test object cannot be seen by the technician or co-worker, it may be necessary to check the construction drawings to determine what is causing such a signal to appear.

Prior to performing angle beam tests, a straight beam test of the scanning surface is generally required by most codes and specifications. The purpose of this scan is to determine that the base metal beneath the angle beam transducer does not contain discontinuities, particularly laminations that might interfere with the angle beam testing. If the base metal is laminated, the sound beam may reflect from the lamination rather than the back wall. If this occurs and is not caught prior to testing, the technician will not have any idea where the sound beam is actually going, rendering any interpretation impossible.

Doubling is a phenomenon that can occur when performing straight beam tests, especially on materials that may be subject excessive thinning from internal erosion or corrosion, such as when testing pipe or tank shells. As the transducer moves onto progressively thinner material, there may be a sudden jump in thickness to approximately twice the previous reading. This is an indication that doubling has occurred.

At this point, the sound reflects from the backwall faster than the transducer can read it, so the first return signal is not seen. The sound then makes another round trip in the material and the transducer picks up the sound on the second round trip through the material, causing the reading to appear to be twice the actual thickness. A simplified example of this shown in Figure 8.27, where good readings are taken at *A*, *B* and *C*, then the reading doubles at *D*, making the material look twice as thick as it actually is.

This problem tends to occur most often when using digital thickness testers with short (or no) delay lines, but can occasionally occur with A-scan units, and usually happens when the materials thickness drops to the 0.15 to 0.2 cm (0.06 to 0.08 in.) thickness range. This range will vary depending on the transducer type, and in some cases the thickness tester can be tuned by the manufacturer to get lower readings, but the best way to eliminate this problem is by using delay line transducers to provide a longer stand-off.

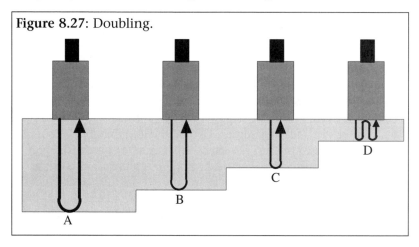

Figure 8.27: Doubling.

Chapter 9

Ultrasonic Testing Applications

INTRODUCTION

This chapter is devoted to the manner by which ultrasonic techniques are used to ensure test object compliance with acceptance criteria, as carried out in several manufacturing and field service environments.

Ultrasonic tests are used for gathering information on test objects made from an array of materials in many configurations. This classroom training book emphasizes industrial and engineering applications where ultrasonic testing is used for materials characterization during manufacture and service.

During fabrication and assembly, ultrasonic testing is used to ensure that an object meets the quality criteria specified in original design specifications. These criteria often require an absence of various types of discontinuities, including cracks, inclusions and voids in specified concentrations or sizes.

During inservice tests, ultrasonic testing is used, along with other nondestructive testing methods, to assess a test object's integrity. The gathered information is coupled with analytical estimates (fitness for service engineering analysis) of the likelihood that the test object will continue to perform its intended service in its current state. Such analysis often involves information such as wall thickness, presence of cracking or other service related damage that can only be gathered by use of ultrasonic testing.

Ultrasonic testing, along with most other nondestructive testing applications, provides information that, when combined with other test date, design criteria and usage history, helps engineers make a judgement as to the ability of the test object to withstand anticipated mechanical loading from applied or residual stresses. These stresses might be static or cyclical. In most cases, nondestructive testing is mandated by safety regulations, as well as economic factors and liability exposure. Its use begins with testing of raw materials used in manufacturing or construction, continues through joining of subcomponents, is part of the quality assurance program and process control activities and continues through the life of the test object, in the form of inservice maintenance tests.

Users of ultrasonic testing for new construction include electrical utilities, petrochemical plants and their pipeline systems, commercial buildings and transportation sectors such as aerospace, auto, rail and marine. Ultrasonic testing is used in evaluating primary and secondary raw materials, formed and machined subcomponents, as well as joints created through welding, brazing and bonding.

The specifications calling for nondestructive testing of new materials and assemblies are based on the specific service environment of the test object throughout its service life. For example, objects exposed to static compressive load are often relatively benign in comparison to those subjected to large, cyclical stresses. The dynamic environment requires that the test object is free of crack inducing discontinuities that can be detected using ultrasonic nondestructive testing.

When applied to field activities, nondestructive testing is used to verify proper installation of major components and to monitor inservice degradation through regular testing cycles, in support of plant and facilities maintenance or upgrading projects. Components are retested at intervals commensurate with projected rates of degradation and support, or sometimes conservative maintenance practices.

The following sections discuss how ultrasonic testing is applied in common industrial applications. The flat surface test is considered first, followed by curved surfaces and highly irregular surfaces. The discontinuities being sought are either planar (two-dimensional) or globular (three-dimensional). Since planar discontinuities exhibit directional reflections, they are further subdivided into orientations parallel and perpendicular to the test surface. Different ultrasonic testing techniques are needed to effectively detect both conditions.

Test Objects with Flat Surfaces

Many objects tested with ultrasonic testing are flat with parallel surfaces. Rolled plate, bar, sheet, flat castings, extrusions, ingots, billets, forgings and engineered materials such as composite and honeycomb panels are among the common ultrasonic test objects. The most common metal forms are wrought metals made into plates and sheet by sequential rolling. Such materials originate from billets and are rolled into strip, sheet, plate and bar. They can contain relatively smooth and flat discontinuities that are either parallel (laminations, debonds) or perpendicular (cracks, lack of penetration, seams, splits) to the major surface of the test object. Castings, forgings and welds can also have internal discontinuities that tend to scatter reflected sound in a random manner (gas pores, slag inclusions, forging bursts, shrinkage, chevron and intergranular cracks).

DETECTING PLANAR DISCONTINUITIES

Planar discontinuities act as smooth, flat reflectors and reflect a strong, clearly defined pulse. When the transducer is properly aligned with the reflected beam, the response is clear and crisp on the A-scan display. If the transducer is not closely aligned with the reflected beam, the reflected beam can be completely missed during a typical test.

Planar discontinuities often have an orientation within a test object based on the manner by which the test object was manufactured or the type of service stress to which it has been exposed. For example, cracks are usually located at the surface of a test object, propagate into the material and may run along a plate or shaft. Similarly, seams and laminations tend to be aligned in the directions of drawing and rolling, respectively.

The strategy in detecting these conditions is to position the transducer so that it introduces the sound beam into the region of interest (surface, full volume, corner) with a beam direction that is perpendicular to the most probable orientation of the discontinuity. Many classes of discontinuities are found using longitudinal ultrasonic waves sent into the test object perpendicular to the surface, so that planar discontinuities that are parallel to the beam entrance surface may be easily detected.

Discontinuities Parallel to the Entry Surface

A major concern in rolled products is the elongation of voids and inclusions into extended laminations or stringers. Dirty steel, for example, contains an excessive number of minor laminations or stringers embedded within the base material. Because of the rolling and drawing processes, these discontinuities tend to be aligned with the rolling direction. Forgings also have discontinuities that tend to be aligned with flow lines. Castings and welds, on the other hand, generally contain more symmetrical reflectors caused by gas pores, local segregation, included bits of slag and local shrinkage. Figure 9.1 shows several variations of discontinuities that can be found in flat test objects.

Laminar discontinuities are detected using longitudinal waves directed through the width of the material. This is the simplest application of pulse echo ultrasonic testing. Strong and consistent signals are reflected, from typical internal discontinuities and from the back surface. The back surface signal serves as a consistent time or location reference. Castings are tested with the same configurations as plates, but discontinuity signals are less pronounced and are more difficult to detect. Figure 9.2 shows the echoes received by the reflectors in Figure 9.1.

For applications involving a single reflector (discontinuity or back wall indications), the ultrasonic testing instrument's display is calibrated so that the front surface indication is on the left of the A-scan display while the back surface echo appears on the right of the display.

This setup is the same for both contact and immersion techniques. Note that the water travel time must be removed using the time delay control for immersion tests. In this case, the spacing between the immersion transducer and the front surface must be slightly more than one-fourth of the thickness of the test object to

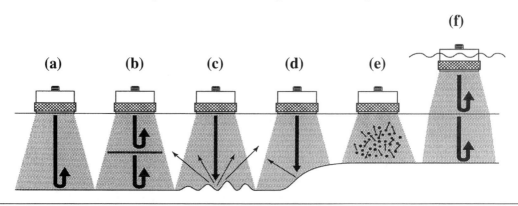

Figure 9.1: Ultrasonic test of parallel reflectors in products with parallel surfaces.

(a) (b) (c) (d) (e) (f)

Figure 9.2: A-scan display for conditions shown in Figure 9.1.

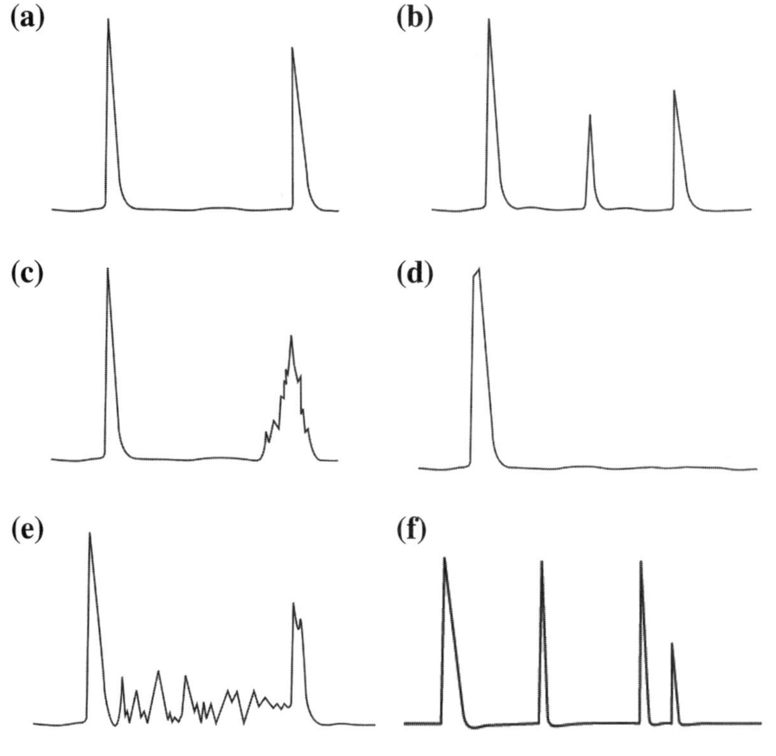

(a)

(b)

(c)

(d)

(e)

(f)

ensure no multiple pulses of the water path occur between the front and back surface pulses from the test object.

Calibration of the horizontal axis is established using multiple reflections within a known thickness of an acoustically similar material. This is done using a calibration block like the International Institute of Welding (IIW) block or a step wedge cut into increments through the thickness range of interest. When lamination detection is performed, the horizontal location of the echo pulse defines the depth of the lamination.

When thickness is being measured, the back surface echo position defines the thickness. This is the primary method used to detect and estimate the extent of internal pipe or tank wall thinning from the outside surface. In general, the time of arrival of pulses within a test object is the most precise measurement an ultrasonic system can deliver.

Since the time of arrival (and not the relative signal amplitude) establishes the relative thickness of a test material, vertical axis calibration is somewhat arbitrary. Thickness measurements can be made as long as a strong signal is reflected from the back surface. As the back surface of materials become increasingly rough, the exact start point of an echo is more difficult to determine, the back wall echo becomes less distinct and thickness measurement becomes less precise.

Calibration of the vertical axis is very important when detecting reflectors of a specific size. The normal approach is to use blocks with precisely drilled holes. Vertical, flat bottomed holes serve as disk shaped calibration targets. Horizontal, side drilled holes reflect sound in the same way as a cylinder. In either case, the target (hole) size is mandated by procedure (or chosen by experience) so that the gain of the ultrasonic instrument is sufficient to display a pulse height of about 80% full screen height or more when a significant discontinuity is encountered.

Gating Applications

For a base material with many discontinuities that scatter the beam (stringers and elongated clusters of inclusions or voids), the acoustic energy reaching the back surface becomes increasingly attenuated. In extreme cases, such as in coarse grained castings, the back surface reflection can be totally absent from the A-scan display. In this situation, two gates are used to monitor the relative pulse heights. One gate monitors the bulk of the test object. The other is triggered by changes (drops) in the back surface signal.

Discrete pulses occurring within a test object indicate the presence of single, coherent internal reflectors. A reduction in the signal received from the back surface indicates that the surface is rougher than usual, the back surface is no longer parallel to the front surface or intervening scattering reflectors exist, even if they cannot be seen as discrete pulses.

The A-scan display for flat plate geometries identifies the location of the front surface, the back surface and the depth of detectable intermediate reflectors. When these clearcut A-scan data are used for constructing a C-scan of the test object, the resulting images can portray the plan view area of internal reflectors as well as the depths at which they exist.

In the simplest case, any echo exceeding a selected threshold amplitude can be regarded as the location of a significant discontinuity. The gate used for this purpose starts just behind the front surface indication and ends just in front of the back surface indication. The resulting C-scan image displays, at a minimum, two levels of density or possibly color. The one density or color represents the surface areas where no reflectors are detected. The other density or color represents areas where reflectors have detected with the threshold setting of the gate.

A more complex gate, or a system capable of advanced signal processing, captures the time delay or time of flight between the start of the gate and the time when the internal reflector pulse is detected. Deeper reflectors produce longer time delays. In this case, the C-scan portrays both the locations where reflectors are detected and their relative depth below the test object surface. This depth information is portrayed by assigning a different density or color to each delay time increment. A reflector near the top surface can be made to appear dark or of a specific color on the C-scan, while a deeper reflector appears lighter or of another color.

It is important to remember that a smaller reflector located in the shadow of another larger discontinuity may not be detected at all. Depending on its size relative to the sound beam's cross-sectional area, most ultrasonic pulse energy is reflected from the first discontinuity it encounters, effectively masking other reflectors located behind it.

Another effect that may be observed is the introduction of multiple reflections between a test object's top surface and a parallel reflector near the surface. Such multiple pulses display a typical ring-down pattern that appears as a periodic series of indications within the body of the test object. The successive echoes are not each a new defect, but simply echoes of the original defect. They are displayed as equally spaced striations within a B-scan (cross-section) display of the test object.

The Special Case of Thin Materials

Thin gaged materials, such as sheet and composites, are usually tested with longitudinal wave transducer configurations similar to those used with plates. However, higher near surface resolution and different interpretations of the A-scan displays are sometimes necessary. The problem with thin materials is that ultrasonic systems may not be able to clearly discriminate between the front and back surface, even when used at the instrument's best depth resolution settings. When using contact transducers, the region of interest is well within the near field and consistent results may not be possible.

One approach is to move the transducer away from the surface of the test object using a spacer such as an acrylic rod. Figure 9.3 illustrates a single element probe that is attached to an acrylic rod standoff. Such a standoff transducer design positions the test material in the far field, where the sound pattern is uniform but a large interface signal still occurs at the surface of the test object.

Figure 9.3: Standoff attached by use of threaded fitting that joins the transducer face to an acrylic rod. (Coupling agent is used between the transducer and rod, and between the rod and test object.)

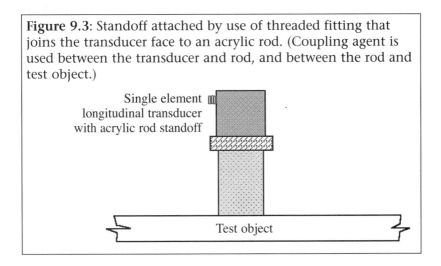

On the A-scan display using a single element transducer, multiple reflections from a thin walled test object can make detection of a discontinuity difficult. A dual element transducer, with one element serving as a transmitter and the other functioning as a receiver, provides a representation of the sound wave/material interaction that is much easier to interpret. Some dual element transducers have the elements mounted side by side and slightly inclined toward each other, as shown in Figure 9.4. The region where the refracted waves intersect within the test object is a zone of higher detection sensitivity and exhibits a greatly enhanced sensitivity to reflectors with surfaces that are parallel and near the surface of the test object.

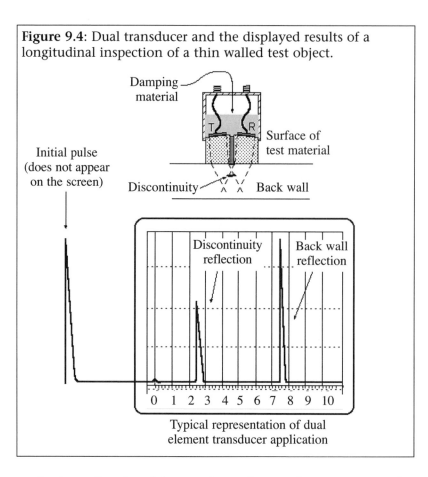

Figure 9.4: Dual transducer and the displayed results of a longitudinal inspection of a thin walled test object.

Damping material

Surface of test material

Initial pulse (does not appear on the screen)

Discontinuity

Back wall

Discontinuity reflection

Back wall reflection

0 1 2 3 4 5 6 7 8 9 10

Typical representation of dual element transducer application

As the roof angles of the transducer elements become steeper, the region of sensitivity moves closer to the surface. Its sensitivity also becomes more pronounced. Reflectors in this region are detected while deeper reflectors are most likely to be missed. The dual element transducer is a setup that works well for thickness gaging within a relatively narrow range of depths. The signal response is enhanced by the absence of a strong echo from the entry surface. One problem is a small amount of leakage across the bottom of the acoustic barrier between the transmit section and the receive section, but this is minimal in most cases.

For finding discontinuities parallel to the test surface in thin sheet materials, another technique uses the array of reverberations that result from sound bouncing within the homogeneous layers of the sound path. This is shown in Figure 9.5. The resulting types of signals are shown in Figure 9.6b and 9.6c for a spot weld like that shown in Figure 9.6a. A well fused spot weld yields the pattern shown in Figure 9.6b, while an unfused spot weld looks like Figure 9.6c. The unfused weld yields a pattern of pulses that is spaced about half of that expected for a good weld. The general shape of the secondary (or lower amplitude) pulses in the unfused pattern tends to grow in amplitude rather than decay. This apparent doubling of

Figure 9.5: Ultrasonic echoes from spot weld coupons [the principle echoes in (a), (b) and (c) are spaced out 0.48 µs apart in two layers of 0.07 cm (0.028 in.) welded steel]: (a) good weld; (b) undersize weld; (c) stick weld; and (d) no weld.

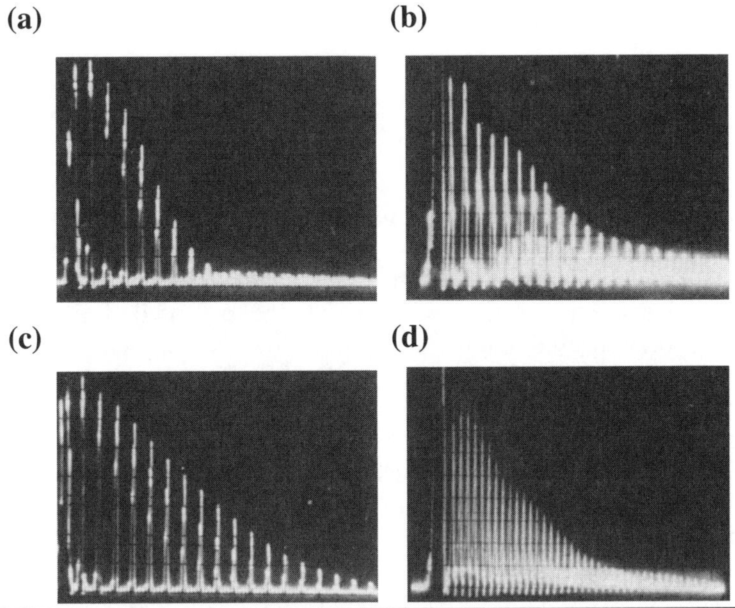

(a)

(b)

(c)

(d)

Figure 9.6: Ultrasonic pulse echo spot weld test: (a) wave paths in satisfactory weld; (b) echoes from the satisfactory weld; (c) wave paths in an undersized weld; and (d) echoes from the undersized weld.

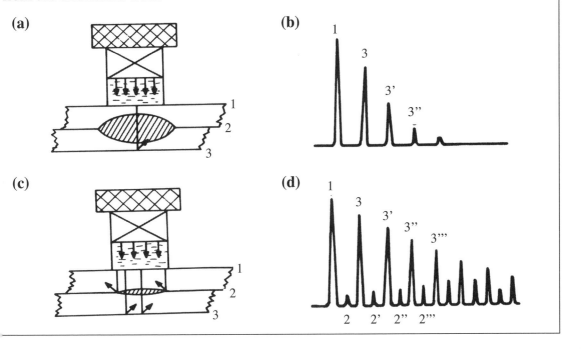

(a)

(b)

(c)

(d)

pulses and partial growth is the indicator the test object is not homogenous throughout its thickness.

This same technique is used when thin sheets of metallic materials are bonded or brazed together. The pattern indicates that the acoustic properties are not uniform throughout the thickness of the bonded region. That information alone is usually enough to cast doubt on the integrity of the bonding process. Note that no information is attainable regarding the exact depth of the debond, however a C-scan image will show the location of the separation in this type of interpretation. The basis for creating the C-scan relies on selection of a distinct feature of the ring-down zone that correlates with the debonded conditions.

When testing thin sheets of engineered materials such as graphite epoxy composites, the difficulty lies in assessing the uniformity of acoustic properties, particularly when such materials exhibit excessive scatter and absorption. Composite materials are composed of high strength fibers encased in a weaker matrix. When tested by ultrasound, these materials produce multireflective interfaces that limit the ability of reverberations to occur within the materials themselves. The ring-down effect, seen for metallic sheets, does not work in this case.

Composite materials development laboratories have had success with sound that travels through the material twice. This approach doubles the system's sensitivity to sound impeding voids or delaminations and, in the case of bonded structures, debonded regions. This technique uses what is called a *reflector plate* on the far side of the thin materials tested with an immersion technique. Figure 9.7 shows the setup and a typical A-scan display. The transducer is scanned above the test object in a rectilinear pattern (X versus Y). The resulting C-scan uses the signal drop from the reflector plate echo as the basis for plotting image density differences. When the signal drops below the gate's threshold, the intensity (or color) of the test object's image changes accordingly.

Figure 9.7: Reflector plate technique used with thin composite panels.

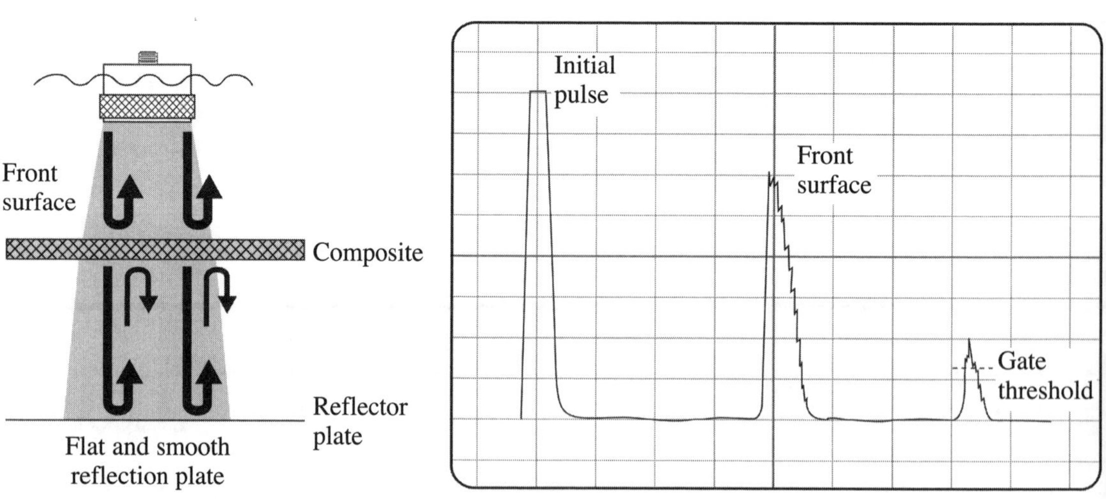

Discontinuities Perpendicular to the Entry Surface

Planar discontinuities, with a principal reflecting surface perpendicular to the surface of ultrasonic wave entry, are not reliably detected with conventional longitudinal wave transducers. These discontinuities include most types of surface connected cracks, as well as lack of penetration and lack of fusion in welds. Unfavorable orientation between beam direction and reflector surface makes these tests unreliable.

Perpendicular planar reflectors are detected using sound beams traveling at relatively steep angles (shear waves) to the entry surface. Shear waves are trapped and sent back from the corners created by the crack and test object surface. This geometry presents the opportunity for incident sound beams to be redirected along the same paths they traveled in reaching the locations of such corner reflectors. This is the concept behind angle beam shear wave pulser/receiver transducers.

Cracks are mostly associated with free surfaces and tend to grow inward (away from the surface) as well as along the surface. Although they may have somewhat different detailed surface morphologies, they are ideal for detection with angle beam testing techniques.

Since cracks are mostly initiated from a surface, one might think that surface wave ultrasonic techniques would work best for this kind of crack detection. Unfortunately, surface waves are restricted to a depth that is limited by the sound's wavelength. Surface waves are also very sensitive to surface conditions, such as roughness and the presence of sound damping liquids. For these reasons, surface waves tend to be used only on smooth, dry surfaces that are not flat. Since a surface wave will follow an undulating contour, they are sometimes used on gently changing shapes such as turbine blades and vanes.

For materials with generally parallel surfaces, such as plate and pipe, the sound beam can be reflected from the parallel surface to redirect the beam toward the entry surface. A shear wave transducer, as shown in Figure 9.8, is used for contact testing. Figure 9.9 shows the same concept used in the immersion technique for both plate and heavy walled pipe. In either technique, the incident sound beam is angled within the test object. Reflected echoes from surface connected cracks travel back toward the sending transducer.

Because the reflecting cracks are at some distance from the transducer, the orientation of the transducer is critical. Rotation of the transducer by only a few degrees is enough to completely lose the echo signal, particularly if more than a single bounce is used.

This angle beam approach is the primary way cracks are detected in and around welds. It does not have the convenience and comfort of the simple thickness mode (used for laminations) because no consistent back surface reference signal is present. A signal is received only when the sound beam is reflected from a discontinuity or some other geometrical reflector, such as a corner at the plate's

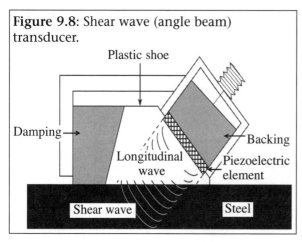

Figure 9.8: Shear wave (angle beam) transducer.

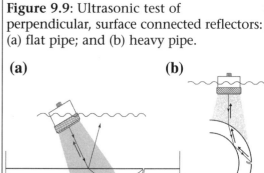

Figure 9.9: Ultrasonic test of perpendicular, surface connected reflectors: (a) flat pipe; and (b) heavy pipe.

end or the crown or root area of the weld. The A-scan interpretation is further complicated since the location of the transducer, with respect to the weld, changes during scanning.

With no consistent reference reflector and various portions of the beam being used, the integrity of the testing process depends on a careful calibration process. The precise beam angle and exit (or index) point must be known and the horizontal sweep must correlate accurately with the actual sound path within the test object.

Figure 9.10 shows how echoes from surface breaking cracks occur at different locations across the A-scan display. As the transducer is moved away from the weld, the beam passes through the center of the weld, intersects the root of the weld and eventually encounters the crown of the weld. Signals appear on the display only when the transducer is positioned at a location where an echo pulse is reflected along the original path of the incident beam.

Since the discontinuities of interest can be several inches from the transducer, the signal fall off with distance must be considered and a distance amplitude correction scheme must be incorporated into signal interpretation. The shape of the distance amplitude correction curve may be drawn on the A-scan screen (either physically or electronically) to serve as a reminder of the degree to which the signal amplitude falls off with increasing distance. If the ultrasonic testing instrument is equipped with programmable gain compensation, an electronic distance amplitude correction increases the gain with increased distance, so that the displayed pulses appear to have the same height regardless of the reflector's distance from the transducer.

Figure 9.10: Weld testing using contact shear waves that intersect: (a) the weld center; (b) the weld root; and (c) the weld crown.

(a)

(b)

(c)

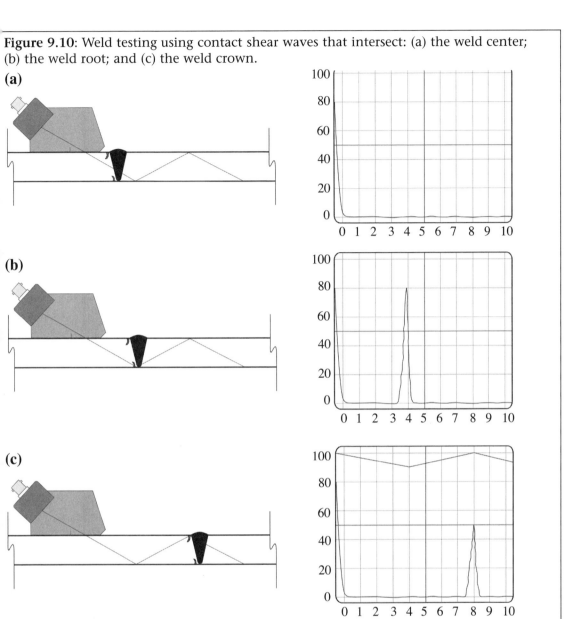

Discontinuities Removed from Entry Surface

Planar discontinuities that are removed from accessible surfaces include lack of sidewall fusion and incomplete penetration in double-vee welds. Such discontinuities are often difficult to detect because of their poor orientation to the pulse echo transducer. In some cases, they can be detected based on a predetermined orientation with respect to weld geometry. For example, the double-vee weld shown in Figure 9.11 has its root near the midthickness region of the weld. If conventional angle beam shear wave testing is used, the reflection from the discontinuity (lack of penetration) would not return to the transducer. However, a second receiver can be used, as shown in Figure 9.11, to detect signals reflected from the face of the root preparation zone. As long as the root area is filled with weld metal, no signal will be received by the receiver transducer.

Lack of sidewall fusion occurs on the right side of the weld in Figure 9.11. A pulse echo transducer is able to detect this discontinuity with a beam that intersects the weld preparation surface at right angles. The incident beam must be perpendicular to the fusion line to reliably detect lack of sidewall fusion.

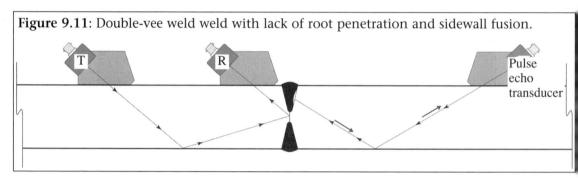

Figure 9.11: Double-vee weld weld with lack of root penetration and sidewall fusion.

SCATTERING DISCONTINUITIES

Planar discontinuities are noteworthy because of their directional reflectivity patterns. Scattering discontinuities (voluminous and globular) tend to scatter incident sound beams into many directions without the highly preferential directionality found with planar reflectors. Examples include gas pores, irregularly shaped inclusions and shrinkage found in castings and welds, as well as bursts in forgings and chevron cracks found in drawn bar. This class of reflectors is relatively easy to detect in fine grained metallic structures.

The scattered nature of the reflections is caused by both the overall geometry and the irregular surface of the scattering discontinuities. Since they do not reflect a strong single echo, their indications on an A-scan are smaller and less distinct than those obtained from properly oriented planar reflectors. However, the scattered nature of the reflections permits detection from numerous vantage points, so that sending and receiving pairs of transducers can be used for locating such scattering discontinuities. Careful alignment of the transducer is not necessary when testing for these reflectors.

TEST OBJECTS WITH CURVED SURFACES

Ultrasonic testing of objects with simple curved surfaces (shafts, tubes and pipes, castings and forgings) is generally done with techniques that compensate for test object curvature. The major problems are: maintaining consistent coupling; stabilizing transducer rocking motions (while scanning); and compensating for the defocusing and distorted effects the curved surface creates in the sound beam. Test objects with a small radius of curvature are more troublesome than the larger diameter test objects.

For example, a large diameter welded pipe is tested using the same setups used for flat plate butt joints. However, as the diameter drops below 50 cm (20 in.), the curvature of the surface causes the couplant across the face of the contact transducer to become nonuniform. The transducer is also subject to rocking during scanning. In addition, the curvature of the test object, acting as an acoustic lens, diverges the sound beam within the pipe. As the size of pipe decreases, these effects become increasingly pronounced.

To stabilize the mismatch of the flat transducer and the curved test object, a conforming plastic shoe can be used. Although this technique makes coupling uniform and controls transducer rocking, it also inhibits rotation of the transducer and does little to correct beam divergence.

Correction for beam divergence can be achieved by using a contour correcting lens for immersion testing. In the case of contact testing, a special curved piezoelectric element is needed to serve the same purpose, with a different shoe and transducer element for each pipe diameter or curvature.

TEST OBJECTS WITH IRREGULAR SURFACES

The most challenging applications for ultrasonic testing are objects with highly irregular shapes. Examples include nozzles used to join piping to heavy wall vessels, turbine and jet engine disks and blades, and large tube intersections in K or Y configurations. All of these are tested using ultrasonic techniques, but extreme care must be taken in positioning and manipulation of the transducers.

Curved surfaces can often lead to internal mode conversion of the ultrasonic wave in objects other than welds, which were discussed previously. This complicates interpretation of the signals, as shown in Figure 9.12. The longitudinal transducer at the left, positioned to test the length of the axle, inadvertently creates a mode converted shear wave at the reflection point T, caused by a fillet in the shaft. The transverse wave moves along the axle, mode converts to a longitudinal wave and eventually returns to the sending transducer. The elapsed time would suggest that a transverse discontinuity might be located in the axle at the false reflection site.

> **Figure 9.12**: Typical false echo path caused by a reflected transverse wave at the axle fillet and a reflected longitudinal wave on the opposite side.
>
> Reflection point T Reflected longitudinal wave
>
> Incident wave
>
> Bearing housing
>
> Apparent location of false indication
>
> Transducer
>
> Reflected longitudinal wave   Wheel seat   Reflected transverse wave

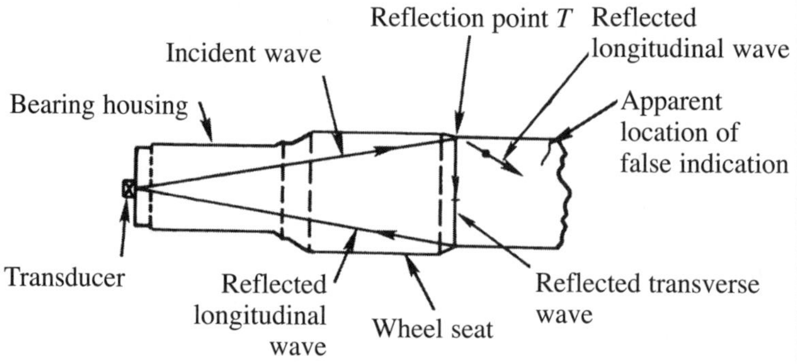

For irregularly shaped test objects such as nozzles, the test is only viable when a specific local region and a specifically oriented reflector are being considered.

A near root condition found in circumferential welds in nuclear piping systems also can create false indications caused by test object geometry. In some pipe welds, a counterbore is used to even the alignment of the two sides of the joint by grinding away enough material in the inner radius of both pipe sections to ensure proper alignment throughout the circumference of the joint. If this ground counterbore is placed too near to the root of the weld, internal reflections can be generated, including some mode converted waves, that are observed when testing for intergranular stress corrosion cracks. Such cracks are generally poor reflectors of ultrasound and ultrasonic testing system sensitivity is quite high, leading to indications from stray reflections coming from the weld root area. Figure 9.13 shows the counterbore geometry and general location of the stress cracks.

> **Figure 9.13**: Typical weld configuration showing intergranular stress corrosion cracking and counterbore.

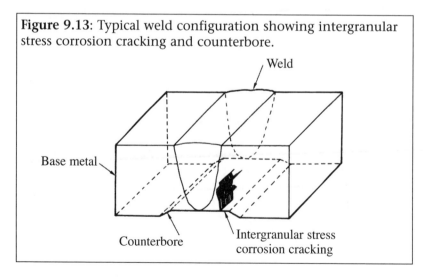

> Weld
>
> Base metal
>
> Counterbore   Intergranular stress corrosion cracking

When two pipes are joined at angles other than right angles, this problem becomes even more pronounced. The Y and K connections have a weld geometry and a test geometry that changes dramatically as the technician follows the path of the fusion zone. The recommended approach for these configurations is use of a properly angled transducer in the very limited area where the beam path is traversing the region of interest. When the access position is changed, the transducer and calibration setup must be reestablished for the new test zone. Another approach demands the use of 45°, 60° and 70° angle beam transducers for the entire weld circumference.

COMPRESSED DISCONTINUITIES

The physical principles of ultrasound predict that a sound beam will be reflected when it encounters a discrete change in acoustic impedance within a material. An air filled crack within a steel plate makes an excellent reflector. However, if the crack surface is smooth and it is under compressive stress, part of the sound will pass through the interface because of the intimate contact and partial deformation of the crack's joining surfaces.

Under extreme pressures, such smooth surfaces may become transparent to an ultrasonic wave with a typical wavelength of about 0.13 cm (0.05 in.). This condition often occurs in the case of press fit cylinders such as bearings and retaining rings in turbine power rotors. Such a joint with a loose fit reflects an ultrasonic pulse, while the same joint under sufficient stress allows the sound to pass through.

A similar condition occurs in the case of a double-vee weld. The smooth walls in the root area of the joint preparation become abutted during the welding operation caused by compressive stresses from shrinkage within the bulk of the weld. When the root pass is not made adequately, the compressive stresses can compress the faces in the root zone so tightly that a shear wave may pass through the joint undisturbed.

Compressed cracks, if detected, can cause other differences in test indications. An open crack may be detected using ultrasound, but sizing can be in error in the presence of high levels of compressed stress. Such stress may be caused by residual stresses, as in the case of the double-vee weld, or by external loading, such as a vertical column or bridge member.

Material Characterization

The acoustic nature of a test object has a pronounced effect on how ultrasound passes through it. Fine grained elastic materials found in many metals are considered homogeneous (same material throughout) and isotropic (same characteristics along all axes). For this class of materials, a sound beam's direction and behavior is highly predictable. These are the attributes assumed in most of the discussions related to detecting and sizing discontinuities using ultrasonic testing techniques.

When ultrasound is used on materials that deviate from these assumptions, the direction a beam takes and the rate at which its energy dissipates is largely dependent on the makeup of the material. These characteristics tend to be cumulative as a beam passes through the material, so that signal strength continues to drop as a beam travels further.

Two conditions predominate in their effects on ultrasonic testing. The first condition relates to the size of partial reflectors that may exist throughout the material. Products such as castings tend to have large grain structures and this scatters the energy of a coherent sound wave. The effect becomes more pronounced as the average size of the grain approaches the wavelength of sound in the material. The result is an increasingly rapid decay in signal strength with distance, a behavior known as the *attenuation of the sound wave*.

The second condition that affects ultrasound transmission involves redirecting the sound path in preferential directions established by the material's anisotropic makeup. In metals, this condition often occurs because of preferential grain growth, particularly in cast stainless steel materials. The presence of both isotropic equiaxed and anisotropic columnar microstructures can be seen in the photomicrograph of a centrifugally cast stainless steel shown in Figure 9.14.

Because ultrasound reacts to different material conditions, such reactions can be used to estimate variations in grain size, density or compactness, age hardening and toughness. Variables used to assess these conditions are usually velocity of ultrasonic wave propagation or wave attenuation.

Figure 9.14: Photomicrograph of centrifugally cast stainless steel showing anisotropic grain structure.

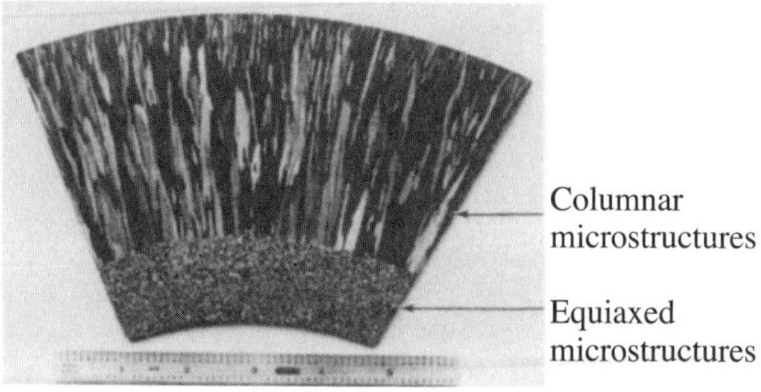

Columnar microstructures

Equiaxed microstructures

Limited Access Tests

In most discussions involving ultrasonic testing, it is often assumed that access is unrestricted, giving total freedom in the placement and angulation of transducers. In many applications, as in the case of the K and Y joints, the geometry of the test object interferes with transducer placement and alignment. For simple geometries like billets, rods, plate, sheet and extrusions, limited access is not a problem. In complex assemblies, the testing plan may call for partial tests of components as the product is assembled because portions of the finished product will not be accessible when assembly is complete.

Limited access is a primary concern when inservice tests are planned. Thermal insulation must be removed, underground pipelines must be exposed, turbine blades at specific locations may be obscured by vanes or support structures. In some cases, complexity of a joint configuration can make traditional ultrasonic testing impossible.

SUMMARY

This chapter addressed the detection and characterization of discontinuities in raw materials and finished components. Test objects with simple and regular geometries (plate, sheet, billets) and curved test objects, such as pressure piping or pressure vessels with large radii of curvature, are relatively straightforward to test. Reflectors parallel to the ultrasonic testing surface are most easily detected, while planar reflectors with varying orientations to the test surface are the most difficult to detect and characterize.

It is the discontinuities – their shape, size and orientation – in a particular material and in a particular environment that determines the technique to be used in their detection. Often, the most challenging task for the nondestructive testing technician is to determine the best technique or combination of techniques for specific test object geometries and suspected discontinuities.

Chapter 10

Transducer Characteristics

INTRODUCTION

Ultrasonic transducers, though identical in appearance and manufactured to the same specification, usually have individual characteristics. Acoustic anomalies may exist because of variations in crystal cutting, areas of poor bond to lens or backing and misalignment of parts in the transducer assembly.

General Equipment Qualifications

Specialized wideband transmitting and receiving equipment is required to accurately measure transducer variables. In analyzing transducer characteristics, the crystal is excited by a voltage spike that will not distort the natural mode of operation. The return signals received by the transducer are amplified without distortion and are displayed in a manner that will provide a permanent photographic record.

The pages that follow describe the special instrumentation equipment and techniques required for measuring, or calibrating, and recording transducer characteristics, such as frequency, sensitivity damping factor, beam size, beam symmetry and beam focal distance.

General Performance Techniques

In general, the transducer calibrating technique consists of scanning a small reflector (a ball bearing, flat post or thin wire) in an immersion tank. As the transducer is moved over the reflector, a changing response that represents a distance amplitude plot of the beam in profile is produced on a display screen. At the highest amplitude portion of the beam, the return signal waveform is photographically recorded when the transducer is held stationary. The waveform is then analyzed to obtain information relating to the frequency, damping ability and sensitivity of the transducer unit.

Using precision manipulative equipment, the transducer is moved over the target and dynamic recording of the beam symmetry is obtained by use of an open shutter camera. These recorded measurements are used in specifying transducers to be used for testing objects that are more uniform.

TRANSDUCER CHARACTERIZATION EQUIPMENT

Equipment used to measure the sending and receiving characteristics of an ultrasonic transducer is capable of reproducing an exact indication on the display screen of the signals sent and received by the transducer. The movement of the transducer over the reflector is accurately controlled. With data potentiometers coupled to sense the motion, a distance amplitude plot of the sound beam is produced on the display screen. An open shutter camera can then be used to record the beam profile on self developing film.

Test Setup

The transducer is placed in a couplant tank made of plastic or glass so that the immersed transducer and reflector can be viewed through the couplant. The reflector is scanned by the sound beam with accurate motion of the scanning transducer ensured through milling table cross feeds to move the transducer. Potentiometers coupled to the cross feeds convert motion data into electrical signals that are fed into the horizontal position controls of the sweep display circuit. The horizontal display shows the distance of transducer traverse in inches. Either X or Y directions of crystal movement are produced by switching from the output of one potentiometer to the output of the other.

Function

Figure 10.1 is a block diagram of instrumentation equipment. The equipment consists of a timer, delay unit, pulser and wideband receiver. The unit repeatedly pulses the transducer with a sharp spike, and then amplifies the return signals fed back through the transducer during operation. Coordination of this activity is performed by the timer (or clock) circuit. The timer triggers both the delay unit and the pulser that later triggers the display circuit.

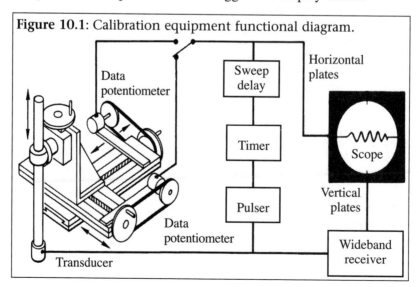

Figure 10.1: Calibration equipment functional diagram.

Recording Method

Figure 10.2 shows how the response curve is recorded with an open shutter camera. The sweep delay, as shown, is used to delay the presentation across the display screen. By this method, a permanent record of the response curve is produced, calibrated in thousandths of an inch, describing the uniformity of the sound beam. This information is related to specific abnormalities in the transducer, such as variations in damping, crystal thickness, lens composition and dimensional nonuniformity.

Figure 10.2: Camera recording method.

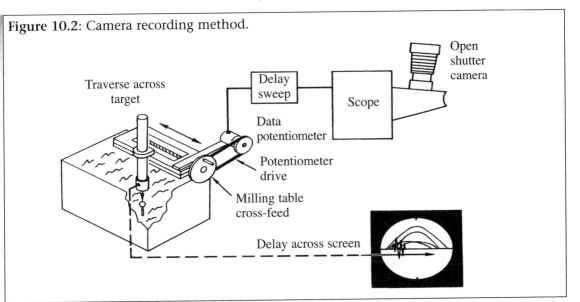

Manipulative Equipment

To obtain precise sound beam and focal length measurements, precision elevating and transversing mechanisms are required. Milling table cross feeds consisting of heavy micrometer screw slides calibrated in thousandths of an inch are used. Two of the slide screws are fitted with sprocket and chain drives connected to data potentiometers that develop the sweep signal.

By relating the micrometer reading to the distance, the trace has moved across the display screen and the recording is calibrated in inches per display division. The two data potentiometers, one on the transverse and one on the longitudinal movement, are provided so that one plot can be made across the target and then, by switching to the other potentiometer, a plot rotated 90° from the first plot can be made. Thus, two recordings of the beam profile can be made without turning or disturbing the mounting of the transducer.

Reflector Targets

Reflector targets must be carefully chosen; a bad target will seriously distort the signal and will produce invalid information. In most cases, precision steel balls are used, particularly when calibrating focused transducers. The diameter of the ball must be as small as possible. The size of the effective reflecting surface of the ball is held to less than one quarter wavelength of the transducer frequency to prevent frequency distortion and undue influence of the target on the measurement of the beam. When analyzing larger diameter flat transducers, a ball target may not offer adequate return signal amplitude for profile recording. In that case, a flat topped post is used as small in diameter as possible. The transducer must be held perpendicular to the flat top surface when testing. Best results are obtained from ball reflectors because they eliminate the difficulty in holding the transducer normal to the flat surface.

Selection of ultrasonic reflectors varies with the geometry of each crystal and lens. Reflectors must be small compared with the beam size measured and about equal in size to actual discontinuities the transducer is expected to detect. For example, a flat, circular reflector of one-eighth the crystal diameter is adequate for testing flat disk transducers used to detect fairly large discontinuities. Spherically focused transducers, used to detect very small areas, produce sound beams much smaller than those produced by unfocused transducers; reflector size is small in proportion. In one experiment, the sound beam traversed a 0.003 cm (0.001 in.) diameter ball taken from a fine line ballpoint pen.

Pulser

The transducer test requires a pulser with a short pulse capability. To analyze the natural frequency and the damping characteristics of the transducer, the transducer must be excited with a voltage pulse that will not drive the crystal into any abnormal oscillation. This requirement demands that the pulse duration be as short as possible, much less than one period of the natural resonant frequency of the crystal.

For analysis of high frequency (5 to 25 MHz) transducers, the recommended pulse duration is 0.025 μs with a rise time of 10 ns (a microsecond is one millionth second, and a nanosecond is one billionth second).

Wideband Receiver

To prevent the received signal from becoming distorted, a receiver with a wideband radio frequency amplifier is used. A recommended receiver is one with a bandwidth of 1.5 to 60 MHz, a rise time response of 10 ns and a gain of at least 40 dB.

Display System

An effective display system has sufficient bandwidth and rise time to present the information without distortion. Bandwidth is direct current to 30 MHz with a rise time capability of 0.01 µs. This scope combination offers delay and time base expansion features that are desirable for recording transducer beam profiles.

RECORDING OF TRANSDUCER BEAM PROFILES

Transducer data sheets are prepared for mounting of photographic records and recording of the transducer analysis factors. The following sections describe various methods used to obtain transducer beam profiles.

Flat Disk Transducer Measurements

Figure 10.3 shows a beam profile plot of responses picked up by a flat disk transducer positioned in water over a reflector. The reflector was made from the butt end of a metal drill which was cut and polished flat. The flat end of the drill and the crystal face were held parallel when the transducer scanned over the reflector along the four parallel paths shown. These four beam amplitude profiles (taken with a moving transducer) plus a return signal waveform (taken with a stationary transducer) were recorded on photographs to provide a permanent record of individual transducer characteristics.

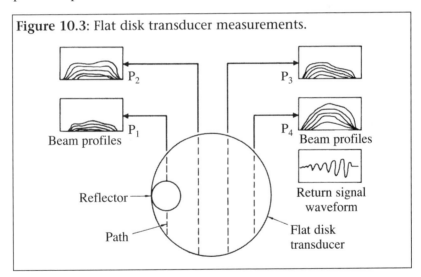

Figure 10.3: Flat disk transducer measurements.

Focused Transducer Measurements

Figure 10.4 shows the basic transducer measurements taken for a focused transducer. With the reflector stationary, a waveform was obtained. Two beam amplitude profile plots were taken with the transducer in the X axis and the Y axis. If the depth of field for moving a focused transducer is required, beam profiles may be taken at points inside and outside the focal point.

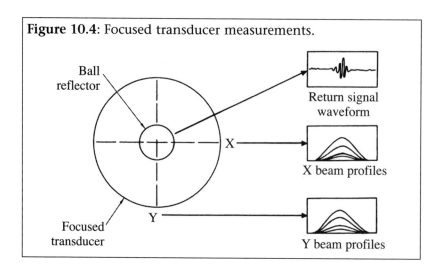

Figure 10.4: Focused transducer measurements.

Cylindrically Focused Transducer Measurements

A wedge shaped sound beam, focused in width and unfocused along the length, is produced by a cylindrically focused transducer that has a concave lens. Beam width is measured by traversing the immersed transducer across the length of the beam over a steel ball reflector, as shown in Figure 10.5.

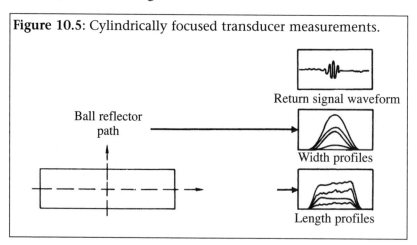

Figure 10.5: Cylindrically focused transducer measurements.

Ball diameter is selected based on the frequency, crystal size and lens radii of the transducer being tested. A rule of thumb is to select as small a reflector as possible that will still produce adequate signal levels for profiling.

Because beam width is usually narrow, the problem of maintaining ball alignment when traversing the beam length may be avoided by substituting a piece of wire for the ball. The wire diameter depends on the same factors that determine ball diameter selection, frequency, crystal size and lens radii.

Two beam amplitude profiles are produced by translating along the beam length over the wire and then translating across the beam width over the ball reflector. The point on the reflector selected for the beam width measurement is determined by the position of the transducer when the beam length measurement is at its point of highest amplitude. With the transducer held stationary, the waveform is also recorded at this point. If the depth of field for the focused area of the beam is required, the beam profile is taken with the transducer moved to two points, where the reflector is nearer than the focal point and beyond the focal point.

ANALYSIS OF TRANSDUCER DATA

In the following sections, each of the main headings on a transducer data sheet are discussed. For each transducer tested, the waveform and beam profile plots are analyzed.

Waveform

The return signal waveform is calibrated in millivolts on the vertical scale with time on the horizontal scale to allow a determination of crystal frequency, damping factor and sensitivity.

Frequency

In frequency analysis, the actual frequency of transducer operation is measured and compared to the design frequency. The actual frequency is a measurement of the acoustic wave in the water medium. As this is the frequency of the energy used when testing material, this is the frequency that is recorded. To record the acoustical frequency of the transducer, the first reflected signal from the ball target is analyzed. The frequency may be calculated if the period (time base) is known. Frequency equals the number of complete cycles per unit of time.

Damping Factor

The damping factor is defined as the number of positive half cycles within the pulse that are greater in amplitude than the first half cycle. By counting the number of cycles generated by the crystal when reacting to the reflected pulse, a measure of the damping factor is reached. With this method, the damping factor is essentially a measurement of the time required for the crystal to return to a quiescent state after excitation. The resolution of the transducer is directly related to the damping factor. The smaller the damping factor, the better the ability of the transducer to resolve two signals arriving very close together in a given time.

Sensitivity

Sensitivity is a measure of the ability of the transducer to detect the minute amount of sound energy reflected from a relatively small target. The vertical amplitude of the received signal, calibrated in volts per centimeter, measures sensitivity. With the amplitude and duration of the pulse known and the amplification factor of the wideband receiver known and held constant, sensitivity is measured in volts peak-to-peak, or in decibels with respect to the pulse voltage.

The ultrasonic reflectors used in a test for sensitivity vary with the geometry of the crystal and lens. In general, the reflector is small compared to the beam size (roughly equal in size to actual discontinuities the transducer is expected to detect). For flat, straight beam transducers, a flat, circular reflector of one-eighth of the crystal diameter is adequate. Beam sizes of focused transducers used to detect very small discontinuities are much smaller than the beam sizes of flat transducers, therefore the reflector is also smaller.

Steel ball diameters ranging from 0.08 to 0.13 cm (0.03 to 0.05 in.) in diameter have been used successfully for testing focused units. These tiny balls are also used for measuring the beam width of cylindrically focused transducers. (These units are focused in the width dimension and unfocused along the beam length.) If difficulties are experienced in aligning the transducer with the ball when traversing along the beam length, a small diameter, fine wire may be laid along the lengthwise path as a substitute for the ball.

Focal Length

The focal length information for focused transducers is the water path distance at which a maximum return signal is obtained. Focal length is the time base measurement on the display screen between the excitation pulse and the point of maximum amplitude response. The transducer is held over the center of the ball target and moved toward or away from the ball until the maximum reflected signal is received. The focal length is then noted and recorded.

Beam Amplitude Profiles

The beam amplitude profiles show amplitude envelopes of each half cycle with the vertical scale calibrated in millivolts of transducer return signal, and the horizontal scale calibrated in mils (or milli-inches) or centimeters of transducer travel. The motion of the transducer across the target drives a data potentiometer that in turn delays the composite signal across the display screen. With the shutter of the recording camera held open, a distance amplitude recording for each individual cycle is produced.

The highest amplitude cycle records the major envelope, the next highest amplitude cycle records the next lower curve, and so on. This recording system produces superimposed response curves from each individual cycle. The symmetry of these curves with respect to one another is indicative of the transducer's operational uniformity in the send and receive modes. The symmetry of these curves is affected by variations in damping, crystal thickness, lens thickness and bonding of the transducer components.

Beam Width and Symmetry

The beam width is read directly from the width of the profile envelope displayed on the calibrated horizontal axis, or at the –6 dB points on each side of the profile peak. Nonsymmetry is recognized as variations in the profile patterns of the propagated sound beam. Through critical analysis of these beam envelope variations, normal and abnormal conditions can be identified. Nonsymmetry may be caused by backing variations, lens centering or misalignment. Porosity in lenses and small imperfections in electrodes and bonding have also been linked to distortion in beam profiles.

Chapter 11

Evaluation Standards

THE ROLE OF STANDARDS IN INDUSTRY

Standardized ways for making and assembling mass produced products came into prominence at the start of the industrial revolution. With the transition from handmade objects to consistent objects featuring interchangeable parts, the stage was set for creating standardized approaches to most industrial activities. Safety concerns also motivated the development of standards, especially after 1900 when catastrophic explosions were common with boilers used in riverboats and public building heating units. Standardization in the United States continued to gain support with the federal government's control of large construction and manufacturing contracts.

In 1898, the American Society for Testing and Materials (ASTM) created a set of standards that addressed the safe construction and use of industrially significant materials including most metals in various grades, ceramics, chemicals, concrete, graphite, paint, textiles, tires and wood. The practices used in nondestructive testing are covered in Volume 03.03 of Section 3, devoted to test methods and analytical procedures. References to these practices can be found throughout the entire set of seventy-two ASTM volumes.

In response to the failures of boilers and pressure vessels, the American Society of Mechanical Engineers (ASME) created the first *ASME Boiler and Pressure Vessel Code* in 1911. As the importance of material quality and integrity of welded joints became evident, the use of nondestructive testing became increasingly prominent in the requirements of the ASME code. Use of the code for construction and testing of nuclear power generation facilities relies heavily on the application of nondestructive testing to detect and evaluate the size of discontinuities throughout the pressure duplication systems.

The American Petroleum Institute (API) was founded in 1919 to standardize engineering specifications for drilling and production equipment. Today, API standards set the criteria for conducting nondestructive testing of piping and storage facilities as well as long distance transmission lines.

The first edition of the *Code for Fusion Welding and Gas Cutting in Building Construction* was published by the American Welding Society (AWS) in 1928. The first bridge welding specification was published separately in 1936. These basic documents have evolved into the *AWS D1.1, Structural Welding Code Steel*, and the *AASHTO/AWS D1.5, Bridge Welding Code*, created to address the specific requirements of state and federal transportation departments.

Such codes and standards are written with a rigorous consensus process using technically competent individuals representing all concerned parties. All of these codes and standards are regularly upgraded to reflect the evolution of technology and the changing needs of user communities. Standards become legally binding when a government body references them in regulations or when they are cited in a contract. Purchasers and sellers incorporate standards into contracts; scientists and engineers use them in laboratories; architects and designers use them in plans; government agencies reference them in codes, regulations and laws; and many others refer to standards for guidance.

Typical Approaches

Ultrasonic tests in a critical or well regulated industry are often covered by multiple documents. For example, the nuclear power generation industry uses procedures written in accordance with the *ASME Boiler and Pressure Vessel Code*. The code, in turn, is supported by published ASTM standards. Sometimes these are augmented by company, customer or Nuclear Regulatory Commission guidelines. To meet the intent of these documents, as well as their stated requirements, testing personnel must assure an employer that ultrasonic testing activities, documented in straightforward procedures, are in compliance with the entire spectrum of applicable codes and standards.

Requirements are stated in codes and standards in ways that differ from document to document. The ASTM standards tend to emphasize the way tests are conducted, but leave the issue of acceptance criteria to be decided by the buyer and the service organization. In this way, the actual testing procedures are left to senior technical personnel, who must agree on an appropriate set of acceptance criteria and related operational issues.

ASME code, Section V sets the ground rules for performing nondestructive testing. However, the extent of coverage, acceptance criteria and interpretation schemes are indicated in other sections, such as those devoted to new construction of power boilers (Section I) pressure vessels (Section VIII), new construction of nuclear components (Section III), and inservice tests of nuclear components (Section XI). The details for testing specific materials are often referred to as *ASTM standards*. To address ultrasonic testing requirements, all applicable sections of the ASME code, including supplemental code cases that clarify specific issues, must be considered.

The issue of safety is so important that most states and provinces within the United States and Canada have written boiler and pressure vessel laws that incorporate ASME codes through direct reference. In these cases, adherence to the ASME code is not just a matter of an agreement between buyers and sellers, but is enforced by the chief technician of the state or province. This legal connection has made ASME code one of the most powerful agents for incorporating nondestructive testing practices into the construction of electric power and processing plants.

In the cases of industry standards like API and ASTM, some latitude is given to the user for establishing acceptance criteria. The basis for final acceptance is usually reflected in the procurement documents but the specific criteria can be altered, provided agreement is reached between the technical representatives of the buyer and the seller. The *AWS Structural Welding Code* also contains such a provision. The AWS code is different from the others in that its cited practices are quite prescriptive, while the others tend to rely more on technician judgment.

The AWS code prescribes transducer sizes, propagation angles and regions within the weld where each transducer is applicable. It sets the compensation for distance in accordance with prescribed near field and beam spread parameters. It prescribes layout markings and protocols for reporting ultrasonic indications. It further defines the classification of indications based on a lookup table that is applicable for either static or dynamic loading.

When still in use, military standards and maintenance technical orders are characterized by their structured approaches based on specific test object configurations and material types. In these cases, the approach to testing is keyed to the particular region in a tested system, with acceptance criteria being based on an accept or reject decision.

Standards and codes may call for interpretation, and their levels of detail may vary considerably. In many organizations, implementation issues are resolved by a team of knowledgeable technical managers who make up what is sometimes called a *materials review board*. It is the task of this board to decide how specific test object conditions are to be processed in compliance with the spirit and directives of an applicable standard or a code.

STRUCTURE OF STANDARDS

Ultrasonic standards tend to identify the approaches allowed for certain tests. They identify how transducers are selected; how scanning is done; when and how calibrations are performed; how to address special situations, such as curved test objects and transfer of calibration data; what acceptance criteria are used; and administrative issues, such as personnel certification and report creation and retention. An ultrasonic test, as cited in some requirements, must address the following items.

1. Instrumentation (selection, operating ranges).
2. Calibration (link to test objects).

3. Search unit type, size and frequency (wave geometry).
4. Screen settings (metal path).
5. Area to be scanned (coverage intensity).
6. Scanning technique (manual, coupling, automatic).
7. Indications to be recorded (minimum sensitivity).
8. Data record format (forms to be followed).
9. Accept/reject criteria (basis or specification reference).
10. Personnel qualifications (certifications).

The degree to which these and other items are controlled is usually dependent on the criticality of the application. Nuclear and aerospace criteria tend to be most demanding, while testing of raw materials is less demanding.

SAMPLE SPECIFICATIONS

Outlined below are excerpts from commercial and military specifications. They are given here to provide an overview of their contents. These excerpts are not complete and should not be considered as replacements for the original issue of a standard. Note that some grammatical and typographical changes have been made for this *Personnel Training Publication*. Contrary to ASNT publications department style, the use of SI units have not been included, as they are not used in the original versions of the following sample outlines.

ASTM Style Standard

ASTM standards define nondestructive tests in an orderly and technically sound manner, often for specific test objects. The standards are intended for use in many different situations, and the details of operational practice are often left to supplemental contractual agreements between the buyer of test services and the seller of the test services. Some of the requirements serve as recommendations for specific actions or as candidates for specific actions. Alternates may be agreed to by the buying and selling participants.

Following is an excerpt from *ASTM A-609, Standard Specification for Longitudinal Beam Ultrasonic Testing of Carbon and Low Alloy Steel Castings*[1]. It defines a system of reference blocks with flat bottom holes, which can be used as the basis for developing distance amplitude corrections. The reference blocks are also used to establish a reference sensitivity for straight beam test systems for cast steel components. The standard further defines conditions under which tests are to occur (material conditions, scan rates, reporting requirements), but it does not give specific information about recalibration intervals, quality levels or personnel certification. The buyer must include these specifics as supplemental requirements.

ASTM A-609, Standard Specification for Longitudinal Beam Ultrasonic Testing of Carbon and Low Alloy Steel Castings is provided (in addition to *Recommended Practice No. SNT-TC-1A*). It has been adapted for this *Personnel Training Publication* with permission.

Excerpt from *ASTM A-609*

1. **Scope**.
    1.1. This specification covers the standards and procedures for the pulse echo ultrasonic testing of heat treated carbon and low alloy steel casting by the longitudinal beam technique.
2. **Basis of purchase**.
    2.1. When this specification is to be applied to an inquiry, contract or order, the purchaser shall furnish the following information.
        2.1.1. Quality levels for the entire casting or portions thereof.
        2.1.2. Sections of castings requiring testing.
        2.1.3. Any additional requirements to the provisions of this specification.
3. **Equipment**.
    3.1. Electronic apparatus: Pulse echo, 1 to 5 MHz, linear ±5% for 75% of screen height.
    3.2. Transducers: longitudinal wave, 1 to 1 1/8 in. diameter, 1 in. square; prefer 1 MHz beyond 2 in. depth.
    3.3. Reference blocks: flat bottom holes, number 16, distance amplitude curve: 1 to 10 in., cast materials that have a metallurgical structure similar to the castings being tested. Other blocks may be used provided they are proven to be acoustically equivalent to the cast steel. The hole bottom shall be cleaned and plugged. Each block identified. Block specifications: 32 rms, flat/parallel to within 0.001 in., hole diameter 1/4 ±0.002 in., perpendicular within 0.5 h.
4. **Personnel requirements**.
    4.1. The seller shall be responsible for assigning qualified personnel. A qualification record shall be available on request.
5. **Casting conditions**.
    5.1. Heat treat before ultrasonic testing.
    5.2. Surfaces shall be free of interference.
6. **Test conditions**.
    6.1. Each pass of transducer to overlap.
    6.2. Rate less than 6 in. per second.

7. **Procedure**.
   7.1. Adjust sweep to put back wall at least halfway across the cathode ray tube.
   7.2. Mark the flat bottom hole indication height for each of the applicable blocks on the cathode ray tube screen. Draw line through indication marks. Set peak at three fourth screen height. This is the amplitude reference line.
   7.3. Use transfer mechanism to compensate for surface roughness differences. Use back wall reflection from block and casting in same thickness and conditions.
   7.4. Attenuator only control that can be changed during testing. Signals may be increased for visibility, but returned to base level for signal evaluation. Calibration should be rechecked periodically using transfer block as basic reflector.
   7.5. Regions having parallel walls and exhibiting loss of back reflection shall be rechecked and treated as questionable until the cause is resolved using other techniques.
8. **Data reporting**.
   8.1. Total number, location, amplitude and area of all indications equal to or greater than 100% amplitude reference line, questionable areas, testing parameters and sketch showing untested areas and location and sizes of reportable indications.
9. **Acceptance standards**.
   9.1. Criteria for individual castings should be based on a realistic appraisal of service requirements and the quality that can normally be obtained in production of the particular type of casting.
   9.2. Acceptance quality levels shall be established between purchaser and manufacturer.
   9.3. Other means may be used to establish the validity of a rejection based on ultrasonic testing.

ASME Style Standard

ASME has structured its nondestructive testing requirements as part of the *ASME Boiler and Pressure Vessel Code*[2]. This comprehensive set of rules defines the allowable design practices, materials, construction practices, testing approaches and documentation. The code ensures consistent construction of new boilers, pressure vessels and ancillary components including piping systems, containment systems and support systems.

The ASME code is subdivided into sections devoted to specific classes of components (pressure vessels, boilers, piping) and supporting technologies (welding, nondestructive testing, materials). Test objects constructed in accordance with the code often satisfy a multitude of requirements. The following pages include brief excerpts from *Section V (Nondestructive Testing), Article 5: Ultrasonic Testing Methods for Materials and Fabrication*[2], as well as examples of how the referencing section of the *ASME Boiler and Pressure Vessel Code* are used for the introduction of specific requirements. An example of ultrasonic testing of ferritic cast materials was chosen to compare with the ASTM specification and a modified set of requirements of Sections III and V.

The important area of weld testing is included to highlight the use of special purpose calibration blocks (not commercial calibration blocks) and to describe methods of verifying instrument linearity and accommodating test object curvatures.

Excerpt from the *ASME Boiler and Pressure Vessel Code*

This outline describes or references requirements that are to be used in selecting and developing ultrasonic testing procedures for welds, objects, components, materials and thickness determinations. *Section V (Nondestructive Testing), Article 5: Ultrasonic Testing Methods for Materials and Fabrication* is provided (in addition to *Recommended Practice No. SNT-TC-1A*). It has been adapted for this *Personnel Training Publication* with permission.

T-510: Scope

When testing to any part of this article is a requirement of a referencing code section, that referencing code section should be consulted for specific requirements for the following.

1. Personnel qualification and certifications.
2. Procedure requirements and techniques.
3. Testing system characteristics.
4. Retention and control of calibration blocks.
5. Acceptance standards for evaluation.
6. Extent and retention of records.
7. Report requirements.
8. Extent of testing and volume to be scanned.

T-522: Written Procedure Requirements

Ultrasonic testing shall be performed in accordance with a written procedure. Each procedure shall include at least the following information, as applicable.

1. **T-523.1: Test coverage**.
   1.2. 10% overlap of piezoelectric element.
   1.3. Rate ≤ 6 in. per second unless calibrated otherwise.
2. **T-530: Equipment and supplies**.
   2.1. Frequency: 1 to 5 MHz.
   2.2. Screen linearity: ±5% in 20 to 80% range.
   2.3. Control linearity: ±20% amplitude ratio.
   2.4. Check calibration at beginning, end, personnel change and at suspected malfunction.

3. **T-540: Applications**.
4. **T-541: Material product forms**.
   4.1. Plate, forgings, bars and tubular products.
5. **T-541.1: Castings**.
   5.1. When ultrasonic testing of ferritic castings is required by the referencing code section, all sections, regardless of thickness, shall examined in accordance with *SA-609*; supplemented by *T-510, T-520*, as well as *T-541.4.1, T-541.4.2* and *T-541.4.3*
6. **T-541.4.1: Equipment**.
   6.1. Transducer shall be 1.13 in. diameter, 1 in.^{2}, 1 MHz, (others allowed if sensitivity acceptable).
7. **T-541.4.2: Calibration**.
   7.1. Blocks: same material specification, grade, product form, heat treatment and thickness ±25%. Surface representative.
   7.2. Longitudinal wave: per *SA-609*.
   7.3. Method.
      7.3.1 Straight beam per *SA-609*.
      7.3.2 Angle beam 80% peak, side drilled hole distance amplitude curve from block.
8. **T-541.4.3: Testing**.
   8.1. Refer to *SA-609*.
   8.2. A supplementary angle beam test shall be performed on castings or areas of castings where a back reflection cannot be maintained during the straight beam testing or where the angle between the front and back surfaces of the castings exceeds 15°.
   8.3. The requirements for extent of testing and acceptance criteria shall be as required by the referencing code section.
9. **T-541.5: Bolting material**.
10. **T-542: Welds**.
    10.1. Requirements for ultrasonic testing of full penetration welds in wrought and cast materials including detection, location and evaluation of reflectors within the weld, heat affected zone and adjacent material. Covers ferritic products and pipe. Austenitic and high nickel alloy welds covered in *T-542.8.5*.
11. **T-542.2: Calibration**.
    11.1. Basic calibration block.
    11.2. Material: same product form and material specification or equivalent P number grouping. P numbers 1, 3, 4 and 5 are considered equivalent for ultrasonic testing. Test with straight beam.
    11.3. Clad: same welding procedure as the production part. Surface representative.

11.4. Heat treatment: at least minimum tempering treatment of material specification for the type and grade and postweld heat treatment of at least 2 h.

11.5. Curvature: >20 in. diameter considered flat to <20 in. diameter.

11.6. System calibration.

   11.6.1. Angle beam (refer to Article 4, Appendix B).

   11.6.2. Sweep range: 10% or 5% full sweep.

   11.6.3. Distance amplitude correction: 20% per 2dB. Echo from surface notch.

   11.6.4. Straight beam (refer to Article 4, Appendix C).

   11.6.5. Sweep range: 10% or 5% full sweep.

   11.6.6. Distance amplitude correction: 20% per 2dB.

11.7. Frequency.

   11.7.1. Change of system component before the end of the test (series), every 4 h and at personnel change.

12. **T-542.6: Welds in cast ferritic products**.

12.1. Nominal frequency is 2.25 MHz, unless material requires the use of other frequencies. Angle selected as appropriate for configuration.

12.2. Distance amplitude curve is not required in first one half V path in material less than 1 in. thick.

13. **T-542.7: Testing of welds**.

13.1. Base metal should be free of surface irregularities.

13.2. Scan with longitudinal wave for laminations at two times sensitivity.

13.3. Manipulate and rotate longitudinal reflectors perpendicular to weld axis at two times sensitivity over reference level.

13.4. Manipulate transverse reflectors along weld at two times from both directions.

14. **T-542.7.2.5: Evaluation**.

14.1. An indication in excess of 20% distance amplitude curve shall be investigated to the extent that it can be evaluated in terms of the acceptance standards of the referencing code section.

15. **T-542.8.5**: Austenitic and high nickel alloy welds.

15.1. Ultrasonic testing is more difficult than in ferritic materials because of variations in acoustic properties of austenitic and high nickel alloy welds, even those in alloys of the same composition, product form and heat treatment. It may, therefore, be necessary to modify and/or supplement the provisions of this article in accordance with *T-110(c)* when examining such welds.

16. **T-580: Evaluation**.
    16.1. With distance amplitude curves, any reflector that causes an indication in excess of 20% of the distance/amplitude curve should be investigated to criteria of referencing code.
17. **T-580: Reports and records**.
    17.1. A report shall be made indicating welds tested, locations of recorded reflectors with operator identification.
    17.2. Records of calibrations (instrument, system, calibration block identification) shall also be included.

Military Style Standard

Military standards tended to use highly specific instructions for their requirements, including the design and use of calibration blocks, methods of system performance analysis and other operating instructions. Below are adapted excerpts from *MIL-STD-2154* which standardized the process for using ultrasonic testing for wrought metals and products greater than 0.64 cm (0.25 in.) thick.

This military standard was applicable to the testing of forgings, rolled billets or plate, extruded or rolled bars, extruded or rolled shapes and test objects made from them. It does not address nonmetals, welds, castings or sandwich structures. It addresses both immersion (Type I) and contact (Type II) methods for testing wrought aluminum (7075-T6, 2024) magnesium (ZK60A), titanium (Ti-6Al-4V annealed) and low alloy steel products (4130, 4330, 4340), using five acceptance classes. Note that *MIL-STD-2154* was superceded by *SAE-AMS-STD-2154*.

Excerpt from *MIL-STD-2154*

1. **Scope**: detection of discontinuities in wrought metals having cross-section thickness equal to 0.25 in. or greater.
2. **Requirements**.
    2.1. Orders shall specify type of testing and quality class in drawings including identification of directions of maximum stresses.
    2.2. Personnel shall be Level II or Level III.
    2.3. Detailed procedure to be prepared for each test object and type of test. It shall cover all of the specific information required to set up and perform the test.
3. **Detail requirements**.
    3.1. Couplants.
        3.1.1. Immersion (Type I), free of visible air bubbles, use preapproved additives, such as inhibitors or wetting agents.
        3.1.2. Contact (Type II), viscosity and surface wetting sufficient to maintain good energy transmission.

4. **Standard reference block materials**: listed alloys or from the same alloy as the test object, free from spurious indications. To be tested to class AA using immersion, longitudinal wave.

5. **Equipment**.
   5.1. Frequency: 2.25 to 10 MHz, refer to *ASTM E-317*.
   5.2. Gain: ±5% full screen height over full range.
   5.3. Alarm: front surface synchronization.
   5.4. Transducers.
      5.4.1. Longitudinal wave, 0.38 to 0.75 in. diameter.
      5.4.2. Shear wave, 0.25 to 1 in. diameter or length.
   5.5. Manipulators.
      5.5.1. Angular adjustment: ±1°.
      5.5.2. Linear accuracy: ±0.1 in.

6. **Reference standards**.
   6.1. Flat surface: Number 2, 3, 5, 8 flat bottom hole per *ASTM E-127*.
   6.2. Curved surface: R <4 in., special block.
   6.3. Angle beam: IIW, for transducer exit/angle side drilled hole block, rectangular beam hollow cylinder block, pipes.
   6.4. Verification: drawings/radiographs, comparison amplitude plots, linearity plots, surface finish, material certifications.

7. **Testing procedures**.
   7.1. Scan parallel to grain flow up to speeds that found reflectors in base materials and at reference amplitude, angulate to maximize, check high stress regions.
   7.2. Near surface resolution limit for 2:1 signal-to-noise ratio: 0.13 in. for 1 in. range through 0.5 in. for 15 in. range. If failure experienced, test from both sides.

8. **Immersion**.
   8.1. Water path: ±0.25 in. of standardization, maximize water-to-metal interface signal, develop distance amplitude curve if needed, angle transducer 23° ±4° to get shear wave from 45° to 70° in aluminum, steel and titanium. Set primary reference response at 80% full screen height. Set scan index between 50 and 80% of the half amplitude response distance from reference standard.
   8.2. Establish for each transducer used. Establish transfer factor using four points from different locations based on back surface reflections or notches, but only if the response is more or less than the comparable signal from the reference standard, allowable range between 60 and 160% or ±4 dB.

Acceptance Criteria

Discontinuities are evaluated with gain set for 80% full screen height on a reference block with hole diameter equal to the smallest acceptable for the applicable class and with a metal travel distance equal to the reflector depth within ±10%.

For longitudinal wave tests, loss of back reflection exceeding 50% shall be cause for rejection unless caused by nonparallelism or surface roughness. Linear discontinuity length is measured using the 50% drop method.

Figure 11.1 illustrates the evaluation technique. *MIL-STD 2154*, paragraph 5.4.16.2 provides the directions for application of this procedure. It reads, "Linear discontinuities: Estimate the length of linear discontinuities having a signal amplitude, corrected by the transfer technique, which are greater than 30% of the primary reference response or 50% of the distance amplitude curve. Position the transducer over the extremity of the discontinuity where signal amplitude is reduced to 50% of the primary reference response or distance amplitude curve. Move the transducer toward the opposite extremity of the discontinuity until the signal amplitude is again reduced to 50%. The distance between these two positions indicates stringer length. Reject any material or test object with linear discontinuities longer than the maximum allowed in the applicable class."

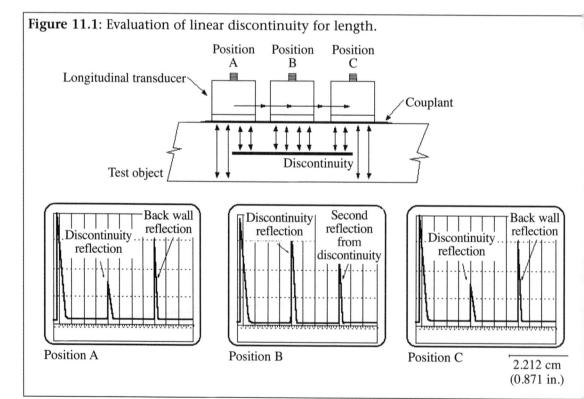

Figure 11.1: Evaluation of linear discontinuity for length.

Quality Assurance Provisions

System performance to be checked before testing, at 2 h intervals during continuous testing, at instrument setting changes or modules and after testing. Distance amplitude curve setups are to be checked daily for the thickness range of material being tested.

Data records shall be kept on file in accordance with the contract. Location and general shape (size) of rejectable indications are to be recorded. Indications in excess of acceptance criteria are permitted if they will be subsequently removed by machining. A C-scan will be made showing the location and size (by discontinuity grade) with respect to the material being scanned.

CONSTRUCTION STANDARDS

Nondestructive testing requirements are often included in the detailed requirements for construction of welded structures that are stressed under static loads (buildings), cyclical loads (bridges) or tubular structures (drilling platforms). Different acceptance criteria are used, based on the purpose of the structure and the types of service to which it is exposed. The base metals are mostly the carbon and low alloy steels commonly found in steel structures.

The criteria listed below are typical for static loading structures. Included are the criteria for rejection, based on different discontinuity classes. Severity is determined by the degree to which the discontinuity indication exceeds a reference level, as modified by sound path attenuation, weld thickness and search unit angle. The classes and reject criteria range from large sizes that are all rejectable to minor discontinuities that are all acceptable.

The presence of more than one class in close proximity is addressed in special notes, as are the treatment of primary tensile stress welds and electroslag welds.

The following sections are representative of a building test code.

1. Personnel qualification: personnel performing nondestructive testing, other than visual testing, shall be qualified in accordance with the current edition of the American Society for Nondestructive Testing *Recommended Practice No. SNT-TC-1A*. Only individuals qualified for Level I and working under the Level II or Level III technician or individuals qualified for Level II or Level III may perform nondestructive testing.
2. Extent of testing: information furnished to the bidders shall clearly identify the extent of nondestructive testing (types, categories or location) of welds to be tested.

SUMMARY

Standards are important for ensuring consistent testing quality in critical industry segments. Their intent is to set a nondestructive testing approach that meets the minimum safety expectations of the user community, yet they must contain sufficient flexibility to be effective for many specific conditions. This level of flexibility is often achieved by letting the supplier and user come to a compromise on specific elements of the standards that apply in a given situation.

When nondestructive testing standards are part of legal requirements for construction and manufacturing, they are often identified in, and used to support, broader based codes. Codes mandate the features of a standard that must be followed and may even be more restrictive than the original standard. The best example of this approach is in the *ASME Boiler and Pressure Vessel Code*, where the product sections (Section VIII for pressure vessels, for example) identify required acceptance criteria, yet testing procedures are found in a separate section (Section V for nondestructive testing).

Many codes reference another set of standards (ASME adopts specific ASTM standards, for instance) or a technical society may reference someone else's code as part of their standard approach to nondestructive testing (API references Section V of the ASME code). Although this approach effectively uses the technical expertise of other organizations, the administration and development of operating procedures for a given company can become complicated. It can be time consuming to compile nondestructive testing application requirements within many of these documents for a particular design configuration. In most standards and codes, the document is setup to first fit material, design and welding needs. Nondestructive testing applications are scattered throughout the text as the primary needs are addressed.

CONCLUSION

The complexity and expense of today's machines and fabricated structures dictate the use of many testing methods and procedures that ensure longer life and function of these machines and structures, as well as the life and health of those who will be working on or close to them. For example, the traveling public is protected every moment of the day by intense nondestructive testing applications applied throughout the body, wing and engine assemblies of all aircraft. Even automobiles are extensively evaluated throughout their assembly by use of various methods of nondestructive testing.

The concepts and techniques that a student and trainee have encountered in this book mark the beginning of an important transition between the introduction to ultrasonic testing techniques and the future of additional instruction, hands on training in the various ultrasonic testing applications and most important on the job experience. Important decisions are made daily based on ultrasonic tests performed by competent technicians, all of whom began their careers as ultrasonic testing students.

With the advent and development of computer interfaced ultrasonic applications, many facets of ultrasonic testing have been made better and easier to use. Yet, human understanding and intuition is still the key element in causing the test systems to generate accurate, trustworthy results.

Glossary

A-scan display: A cathode ray tube or flat panel liquid crystal display in which the received signal is displayed as a vertical height or pip from the horizontal sweep time trace, while the horizontal distance between any two signals represents the material distance (or time of travel) between the two conditions causing the signals.

Acoustic impedance: The factor that greatly influences the propagation of an ultrasonic wave at a boundary interface. It is the product of the material density and the longitudinal wave velocity within the material.

Amplifier: A device to increase or amplify electrical impulses.

Amplitude, echo: The vertical height of an A-scan received signal, measured from base-to-peak or peak-to-peak.

Angle of incidence: The angle between the direction of the transmitted wave and the normal to the boundary interface at the point of incidence.

Angle of reflection: The angle between the direction of the reflected wave and the normal to the boundary interface at the point of incidence. The angle of reflection is equal to the angle of incidence.

Angle of refraction: The angle between the refracted rays of an ultrasonic beam and the normal to the refracting surface.

Angle testing: A testing method in which transmission is at an angle to one test surface.

Angle transducer: A transducer that transmits or receives the acoustic energy at an acute angle to the surface to achieve a special effect, such as the setting up of shear or surface waves in the test object.

Attenuation: The loss in acoustic energy that occurs between any two points of travel. This loss may be caused by absorption, reflection, etc.

Attenuator: A device for measuring attenuation, usually calibrated in decibels (dB).

B-scan display: A screen display in which the received signal is displayed as an illuminated spot. The face of the display screen represents the area of a vertical plane through the material. The display shows the location of a discontinuity as it would appear in a vertical section view through the thickness of the material.

Back reflection: The signal received from the back surface of a test object.

Background noise: Extraneous signals caused by signal sources within the ultrasonic testing system, including the test material.

Barium titanate: (polycrystalline barium titanate). A ceramic transducer material composed of many individual crystals fired together and polarized by the application of a direct current field.

Beam spread: The divergence of the sound beam as it travels through a medium.

Boundary echo: A reflection of an ultrasonic wave from an interface.

C-scan: A data presentation method yielding a plan view through the scanned surface of the test object. Through gating, only echoes arising from the interior of the test object are indicated. In the C-scan, no indication is given of the signal depth.

Collimator: A lens assembly attachment designed to reduce the ultrasonic beam spread.

Compensator: An electrical matching network to compensate for circuit impedance differences.

Compressional wave: A wave in which the particle motion or vibration is in the same direction as the propagated wave (longitudinal wave).

Contact testing: A method of testing in which the transducer contacts the test surface, either directly or through a thin layer of couplant.

Contact transducer: A transducer that is coupled to a test surface either directly or through a thin film of couplant.

Contracted sweep: A contraction of the horizontal sweep on the viewing screen of the ultrasonic instrument. Contraction of this sweep permits viewing reflections occurring over a greater depth of material or duration of time.

Couplant: A substance used between the face of the transducer and test surface to permit or improve transmission of ultrasonic energy across this boundary or interface.

Critical angle: The incident angle of the sound beam beyond which a specific refracted mode of vibration no longer exists.

Cross talk: An unwanted condition in which acoustic energy is coupled from the transmitting crystal to the receiving crystal without propagating along the intended path through the material.

Damping (ultrasonics): Decrease or decay of ultrasonic wave amplitude with respect to time.

Damping (transducer): Limiting the duration of vibration in the search unit by either electrical or mechanical means.

Dead zone: The distance in a material from the surface to the nearest testable depth.

Decibel (dB): The logarithmic expression of a ratio of two amplitudes or intensities of acoustic energy.

Delayed sweep: A means of delaying the start of horizontal sweep, thereby eliminating the presentation of early response data.

Delta effect: Acoustic energy reradiated by a discontinuity.

Diffraction: The deflection of a wave front when passing the edges of an obstacle.

Diffuse reflection: Scattered, incoherent reflections caused by rough surfaces or associated interface reflection of ultrasonic waves from irregularities of the same order of magnitude or greater than the wavelength.

Discontinuity reflection: The screen display presentation of the energy returned by a rejectable discontinuity in the material.

Dispersion, sound: Scattering of an ultrasonic beam as a result of diffuse reflection from a highly irregular incident surface.

Divergence: Spreading of ultrasonic waves after leaving the search unit, a function of material velocity, plus crystal diameter and frequency.

Double crystal method: The method of ultrasonic testing using two transducers with one acting as the transmitter and one as the receiver.

Echo: See **Boundary echo**.

Effective penetration: The maximum depth in a material at which the ultrasonic transmission is sufficient for proper detection of discontinuities.

Electrical noise: Extraneous signals caused by externally radiated electrical signals or from electrical interferences within the ultrasonic instrumentation.

Far field: The region beyond the near field in which intervals of high and low acoustic transmission intensity cease to occur.

Focused transducer: A transducer with a concave face that converges the acoustic beam to a focal point or line at a definite distance from the face.

Focusing: Concentration or convergence of energy into a smaller beam.

Fraunhofer zone: See **Far field**.

Frequency: Number of complete cycles of a wave motion passing a given point in a unit time (1 s); number of times a vibration is repeated at the same point in the same direction per unit time (usually per second).

Fresnel field: See **Near field**.

Gate: An electronic means to monitor associated segment of time, distance or impulse.

Ghost: See **Nonrelevant indication**.

Hash: Numerous, small indications appearing on the display screen of the ultrasonic instrument indicative of many small inhomogeneities in the material or background noise; also referred to as *grass*.

Hertz (Hz): One cycle per second.

Horizontal linearity: A measure of the proportionality between the positions of the indications appearing on the horizontal trace and the positions of their sources.

Immersion testing: A method of testing using a liquid as an ultrasonic couplant in which the test object and the transducer face are immersed in the couplant, and the transducer is not in contact with the test object.

Impedance (acoustic): Resistance to flow of ultrasonic energy in a medium. Impedance is a product of particle velocity and material density.

Indication (ultrasonics): The signal displayed on the ultrasonic screen display.

Initial pulse: The first indication that may appear on the screen. This indication represents the emission of ultrasonic energy from the crystal face, sometimes called the main bang.

Interface: The physical boundary between two adjacent surfaces.

Lamb wave: A type of ultrasonic vibration capable of propagation at specific angles dependent on the product of the test frequency and the test object thickness.

Linearity (area): A system response in which a linear relationship exists between amplitude of response and the discontinuity sizes being evaluated (necessarily limited by the size of the ultrasonic beam).

Linearity (depth): A system response where a linear relationship exists with varying depth for a constant size discontinuity.

Longitudinal wave: See **Compressional wave**.

Longitudinal wave velocity: The unit speed of propagation of a longitudinal (compressional) wave through a material.

Loss of back reflection: Absence of, or a significant reduction of, an indication from the back surface of the object being tested.

Manipulator: A device used to orient the transducer assembly. As applied to immersion techniques it provides either angular or normal incidence as well as transducer-to-test object distance.

Material noise: Extraneous signals caused by the structure of the test object.

Mode: The manner in which acoustic energy is propagated through a material as characterized by the particle motion of the wave.

Mode conversion: The characteristic of surfaces to change the mode of propagation of acoustic energy from one mode to another.

Multiple back reflections: Repetitive echoes from the far boundary of the material being tested.

Nanosecond (ns): One billionth (10^{-9}) of a second.

Near field: A distance immediately in front of a transducer composed of complex and changing wave front characteristics. Also known as *Fresnel field*.

Nonrelevant indication: An indication that has no direct relation to reflected pulses from discontinuities in the materials being tested.

Orientation: The angular relationship of a surface, plane, discontinuity axis, etc., to a reference plane or surface.

Penetration (ultrasonics): Propagation of ultrasonic energy through a test object. See **Effective penetration**.

Piezoelectric effect: The characteristic of certain materials to generate electrical charges when subjected to mechanical vibrations and, conversely, to generate mechanical vibrations when subjected to electrical pulses.

Pitch catch: See **Two crystal method**.

Plate wave: See **Lamb wave**.

Presentation: The method used to show ultrasonic wave information. This may include A, B or C-scans displayed on various types of recorders or cathode ray tube instruments.

Probe: Transducer or search unit.

Propagation: Advancement of a wave through a medium.

Pulse echo method: A single crystal ultrasonic test method that both generates ultrasonic pulses and receives the return echo.

Pulse length: Time duration of the pulse from the search unit.

Pulse method: An ultrasonic test method using equipment which transmits a series of pulses separated by a constant period of time, i.e., energy is not sent out continuously.

Pulse rate: For the pulse method, the number of pulses transmitted in a unit of time. Also called *pulse repetition rate*.

Radio frequency display: The presentation of unrectified signals on a display. See also **video presentation**.

Rarefaction: The thinning out or moving apart of the consistent particles in the propagating medium caused by the relaxation phase of an ultrasonic cycle. Opposite in its effect to compression. The sound wave is composed of alternate compressions and rarefactions of the material.

Rayleigh wave: A wave that travels on or close to the surface and readily follows the curvature of the test object. Reflections occur only at sharp changes of direction of the surface.

Reference blocks: A block or series of blocks of material containing artificial or actual discontinuities of one or more reflecting areas at one or more distances from the test surface, which are used for reference in calibrating instruments and in defining the size and distance of discontinuities in materials.

Reflection: The characteristic of a surface to change the direction of propagating acoustic energy; the return of sound waves from surfaces.

Reflectograph: A recording or chart made of either the signals transmitted through a test object or reflected back from discontinuities within a test object, or both.

Refracted beam: A beam that has been changed both in velocity and direction as a result of its having crossed an interface between two different media and having initially been directed at an acute angle to that interface.

Refraction: the characteristic of a material to change the direction of acoustic energy as it passes through an interface into the refracting material. A change in the direction and velocity of acoustic energy after it has passed at an acute angle through an interface into the refracting material.

Refractive index: The ratio of the velocity of a wave in one medium to the velocity of the wave in a second medium is the refractive index of the second medium with respect to the first. It is a measure of the amount a wave will be refracted when it enters the second medium after leaving the first.

Repetition rate: The rate at which the individual pulses of acoustic energy are generated. Also called pulse rate.

Resolving power (resolution): The measure of the capability of an ultrasonic system to separate in time two discontinuities at slightly different distances or to separate the multiple reflections from the back surface of flat plates.

Saturation (scope): A test indication of such a size as to reach full scope amplitude (100%). Beyond this point, there is no visual display to estimate the actual real height of the response signal unless the equipment is provided with decibel readout.

Scanning (manual and automatic): The moving of the search unit or units along a test surface to obtain complete testing of a material.

Scattering: Dispersion of ultrasonic waves in a medium due to causes other than absorption. See also Diffuse reflection and Dispersion, sound.

Send and receive transducer: A transducer containing two crystals mounted side-by-side separated by an acoustic barrier; one generates the acoustic energy, the other receives it.

Sensitivity: The ability to detect small discontinuities. The level of amplification at which the receiving circuit in an ultrasonic instrument is set.

Shear wave: The wave in which the particles of the medium vibrate in a direction perpendicular to the direction of propagation.

Signal-to-noise ratio: The ratio of amplitudes of indications from the smallest discontinuity considered significant and those caused by random factors, such as heterogeneity in grain size.

Specific acoustic impedance: A characteristic that acts to determine the amount of reflection that occurs at an interface and represents the product of the wave velocity and the density of the medium in which the wave is propagating.

Surface wave: See Rayleigh wave.

Transverse wave: See **Shear wave**.

Through transmission: A test method using two transducers in which the ultrasonic vibrations are emitted by one and received by another on the opposite side of the test object. The ratio of the magnitudes of vibrations transmitted and received is used as the criterion of soundness.

Transducer (search unit): An assembly consisting of a housing, piezoelectric element, backing material, wear plate (optional) and electrical leads for converting electrical impulses into mechanical energy and vice versa.

Transmission angle: The incident angle of the transmitted ultrasonic beam. It is 0° when the ultrasonic beam is perpendicular to the test surface.

Two crystal method: Use of two transducers for sending and receiving. May be send and receive or through transmission method.

Ultrasonic absorption: A dampening of ultrasonic vibrations that occurs when the wave traverses a medium.

Ultrasonic spectrum: The frequency span of elastic waves greater than the highest audible frequency, generally regarded as being higher than 20 kHz to about 100 MHz.

Ultrasonic testing: A nondestructive method of testing materials by the use of high frequency sound waves introduced into or through them.

Velocity: The speed at which sound waves travel through a medium.

Video presentation: A screen presentation in which radio frequency signals have been rectified and usually filtered.

Water travel: In immersion testing, the distance from the face of the search unit to the entry surface of the test object.

Wavelength: The distance in the direction of propagation of a wave for the wave to go through a complete cycle.

References and Bibliography

REFERENCES

1. *ASTM A-609 Standard Specification for Longitudinal Beam Ultrasonic Testing of Carbon and Low Alloy Steel Castings*. West Conshohoken, Pennsylvania: American Society for Testing and Materials International (2000). Reprinted with permission.

2. *ASME Boiler Pressure Vessel Code:* Section V, *Nondestructive Evaluation*. Article 5: "Ultrasonic Testing Methods for Materials and Fabrication." New York, New York: American Society of Mechanical Engineers (2001). Reprinted with permission.

BIBLIOGRAPHY

1. *Nondestructive Testing Handbook*, second edition: Vol. 7, *Ultrasonic Testing*. Columbus, Ohio: American Society for Nondestructive Testing (1991).

2. *Nondestructive Testing Classroom Training Handbook*, second edition: *Ultrasonic Testing*. Fort Worth, Texas: Convair Division of General Dynamics Corporation (1981).

Index

A

attenuation factor, 37, 113
attenuation of sound wave, 15, 164
automatic calibration, 84
automatic mechanical positioning device, 28
auto sector, ultrasonic testing applications, 147
AWS D1.1 Structural Welding Code Steel, 178, 179
AWS standards, 177-178, 179

B

backing bars, 142
backing bar signals, 143-144
barium titanate, 45, 46, 86
    use in through transmission technique, 65
bars
    immersion testing, 90
    MIL-STD-2154, 186
    production, 122-124
    ultrasonic testing, 148
base material product evaluation, 117-146
base material testing, 91-100
basic calibration block, 107-110
beam amplitude profiles, 174-175
beam spread, 51
    Fraunhofer zone, 49
    in steel, 50
beam symmetry, 175
beam width, 175
beryllium
    critical angles of refraction, 22
billets
    immersion testing, 90
    ingots formed into, 117
    limited access tests, 165
    MIL-STD-2154, 186
    pipe and tubular products from, 124
    processing, 120
    ultrasonic testing, 148
bloom, 124
boiler laws, 178
boilers, 178
    ASME standard, 182
bonded (composite) structures, 129-130
bonding, 148, 156
brazing, 148, 156
bridge, in bar and rod production, 123
bridge girders
    high speed scanners for, 68
Bridge Welding Code, AASHTO/AWS D1.5, 178
bridge welding specifications, 177-178

broadband transducers, 85
B-scan display, 25, 27-28, 80, 81-82
bubbler (squirter) technique, 67, 68-69, 90-91
butt welds, 130-131
    angle beam testing, 93
backing bars used with, 142, 144

C

calibration
    equipment, 37-42, 101-116, 167
    instrument standardizing, 37
    standards for, 101, 179
calibration blocks, 37, 38
    for angle beam calibration, 107-116
    area amplitude blocks, 38-39
    ASTM calibration blocks, 40-41
    distance amplitude blocks, 39-40
    IIW reference block, 42
    for straight beam calibration, 104-106
camera recording method, 169
Canada, boiler and pressure vessel laws, 178
carbon steel, 117
casting, 127-129
    continuous casting (concast) process, 118-119
castings
    detecting discontinuities parallel to entry surface, 149
    sample ASME Boiler Code specifications, 183-186
    scattering discontinuities in, 160
    ultrasonic testing applicable to, 4, 148, 161
cast iron, 129
cathode ray tubes, 30
centrifugally cast stainless steel, 164
ceramics
    piezoelectric, 45, 46, 65, 86
    ultrasonic testing applicable to, 4
certification, 7-8
chevron cracks, 148
    as scattering discontinuity, 160
chromium
    added to steel, 117
clock (rate generator), 30, 168
cluster porosity, 128, 140
coarse range control, in pulse echo instruments, 31
Code for Fusion Welding and Gas Cutting in Building Construction, 177-178
codes, 177-179. *See also* standards
    for calibration, 101
    interpretation, 179

and Rayleigh wave mode, 13
    reflection of waves from, 15, 16-17
        removed from entry surface, 159-160
    rod, 122-124
    scattering discontinuities, 160
    slabs and billets, 120
    subsurface, 14
    test objects with flat surfaces, 148
    ultrasonic testing for detection, 3, 4, 76, 147
    welds, 134-142
display/status control, in pulse echo instruments, 32
display system, 76, 77-78, 80-84, 170-171
    pulse echo system, 30
distance amplitude blocks, 39-40, 105-106
distance amplitude correction, 36
distance amplitude correction (DAC) curve
    angle beam calibration, 110, 111
    straight beam calibration, 105, 106
distance corrected gain (DCG), 36
distance sensitivity calibration block, 107, 114-116
documentation, 85-86
double crystal transducer, 64
double submerged arc welding (DSAW), 125
double vee welds, 131, 159
    compressed discontinuities, 163
doubling, 145-146
drawing, 122
dry coupling, 88
dual transducers, 51-52

E

electrical utilities, ultrasonic testing applications, 147
electric resistance welding (ERW), 125
electrodes, imperfections and distortion in beam profile, 175
electromagnetic acoustic transducers (EMATs), 58-59, 61
    other noncontact ultrasonic techniques compared,
        71*table*
electronically focused transducers, 54-55
element, 29
employee certification, 8, 180
energy source, 76
equipment, *See* ultrasonic testing equipment
examination, for certification, 8
experience, 8
external attachment signals, 144-145
extrusion
    of bar and rod, 122
    of pipe and tubing, 124

extrusions, 148
    limited access tests, 165

F

fabrication, ultrasonic testing applications, 147
faced unit transducers, 53-54
far field, 23, 47, 49-50
    beam intensity characteristics, 56
fiber-reinforced plastics
    ultrasonic testing applicable to, 4
fillet weld, 131
fine range control, in pulse echo instruments, 31
first asymmetrical mode, 14, 15t
first critical angle of refraction, 21
    selected materials, 22t
first symmetrical mode, 14, 15t
flat castings, 148
flat disk transducer measurements, 171
flat panel display screens, 30
flexible membranes, mounting over crystal in contact
        testing, 63
flux, 132
flux-cored arc welding (FCAW), 132, 134
flux-cored arc welding-gas shielded (FCAW-G), 135
flux-cored arc welding-self shielded (FCAW-S), 135
foam sandwich panels, air coupled transducers for, 89
focal length, 174
focused beams
    reflector targets, 170
    of ultrasonic waves, 15
    use in immersion testing, 67
focused transducer measurements, 171-173
foreign material inclusions, *See* nonmetallic inclusions
forging, 126-127
    calibration blocks to match amount of hot/cold
        working, 39, 41
forging bursts, 126, 127, 148
    as scattering discontinuity, 160
forgings, 126-127
    detecting discontinuities parallel to entry surface, 149
    MIL-STD-2154, 186
    ultrasonic testing applicable to, 4, 148, 161
fourth symmetrical mode, 15t
Fraunhofer effect, 23
Fraunhofer zone, 23, 47, 49
frequency, 5, 15
    and beam spread, 49, 51
    transducers, 46-47, 49, 84
frequency analysis, 173

frequency control, in pulse echo instruments, 36
Fresnel effect, 23
Fresnel zone, 23, 47
full penetration weld, 130, 131

G

gain control, in pulse echo instruments, 33-34
gases
    longitudinal waves transmit through, 11
    plate, shear, and surface waves don't transmit
      through, 11
gas holes
    castings, 128, 129
gas metal arc welding (GMAW), 132, 134
    discontinuities associated with, 135
gas pores, 148, 149
    scattering discontinuity, 160
    in welding, 140
gas tungsten arc welding (GTAW), 132, 134
    discontinuities associated with, 135
gated alarm units, 36-37
gating, 151-152
glycerin, 62
grain size
    castings, 129, 164
    Lamb wave mode application, 14
graphite epoxy composites, 156
grease, as transducer couplant, 62
groove welds, 130

H

heat, in steel making, 117
heat affected zone (HAZ), 132
high frequency welding (HFW), 125
high resolution transducers, 85
high speed scanners, 68
holes, special calibration blocks, 42
honeycomb structures
    air coupled transducer application, 60
    air coupled transducers for, 89
horizontal base line, 81
hot tears
    castings, 128, 129
    forgings, 126
hydrogen flakes, 123, 124

I

IIW reference block, *See* International Institute of
    Welding (IIW) reference block

immersion coupling, 89-91
immersion tank
    acoustic reflection in, 17
    bar and rod base metal forming, 123
    for immersion coupling, 90
    and near field/far field, 47-50
    transducers in, 167
immersion technique, 67-68
immersion testing, 63, 66. *See also* ultrasonic testing
    couplants, 62, 67
    critical angles of refraction, 21, 22*table*
    detecting discontinuities parallel to entry surface, 149
    and first critical angle of refraction, 21
    first uses of, 4
    and Lamb wave mode application, 14
    techniques, 66-69
impedance, acoustical, 15-16
impedance mismatch, 16
    and couplant selection, 61
impedance ratio, 16
included angle, welds, 131
inclusion laminations, 120-121
inclusions, 147, 151. *See also* nonmetallic inclusions; slag
    inclusions
    castings, 128, 129
    scattering discontinuity, 160
    tungsten, 135t, 142
incomplete penetration, 137, 138, 159
    welding processes associated with, 135
industrial settings, ultrasonic testing in, 86-87
inert gas, in welding, 132
ingots, 117-118
    ultrasonic testing, 148
initial pulse, 80
innerbead lack of fusion, 138, 139
inservice degradation, 148
inservice tests, 147
instrumentation
    calibration, 102-116
    standards for, 179
instrument gain controls, in pulse echo instruments, 31
intergranular cracks, 148
intergranular stress corrosion cracking, 162
internal structure, ultrasonic testing for determining, 3.
    See also discontinuities
internal tears
    pipe and tubing, 125
International Institute of Welding (IIW) reference block,
    42, 102, 107, 150

angle beam calibration using, 111-114

iron. *See also* stainless steel; steel; steel making
  grain size of cast, 129
  production, 117

iron ore, 117

J

jet engine blades, 161

jet engine turbine blades, immersion testing, 90

joints, 148, 161

K

kerosene
  use in early testing application, 4

keypad instrumentation, in pulse echo instruments, 31-32

L

lack of fusion, 137-139, 157
  welding processes associated with, 135

lack of penetration, 148, 157

lack of sidewall fusion, 138, 159, 160

Lamb wave mode, 10, 13-15

Lamb waves, 10

laminated materials
  laser induced ultrasound, 60
  ultrasonic testing applicable to, 3, 76

laminations, 148, 149
  B-scan application for detection, 27
  extruded bar and rod, 122
  pipe and tubing, 125
  plate and sheet, 120-121

laser induced ultrasound, 60-61
  other noncontact ultrasonic technique compared,
    71*table*

lead metaniobate, 46, 86

lead titanate, 45, 46, 86

lead zirconate, 45, 46

lead zirconate titanates (PZT materials), 45, 46

lenses, porosity and distortion in beam profile, 175

Level I personnel
  certification, 7
  examination, 8
  qualification, 5, 6

Level II personnel
  certification, 7
  examination, 8
  qualification, 5, 6

Level III personnel
  certification, 7
  examination, 8
  qualification, 5, 6

limited access tests, 165

linear arrays, 54, 55

liquids
  longitudinal waves transmit through, 11
  plate, shear, and surface waves don't transmit
    through, 11
  sound wave carrier, 10

lithium sulfate, 46, 86
  use in through transmission technique, 65

longitudinal immersion testing, 68

longitudinal wave double crystal transducer, 64

longitudinal wave dual transducers, 52

longitudinal wave mode, 10-11

longitudinal waves, 10
  calculation of refracted angle, 20

longitudinal wave single crystal transducer, 64

longitudinal wave technique, 64

longitudinal wave transducers, 52, 53
  side lobe radiation, 50

low resolution transducers, 85

M

magnesium
  MIL-STD-2154, 186

main bang, 80

maintenance technical orders, 179

manipulative equipment, 169

manufacturing, ultrasonic testing applications, 147

marine sector, ultrasonic testing applications, 147

material calibration control, 31

materials review board, 179

material velocity control, 31

metal inert gas (MIG) welding process, 134

MIG/MAG welding process, 134

military standards, 179, 186
  sample specifications, 186-189
  MIL-STD-2154, 186

mixed mode conversions, 18-19

mode conversion, 12
  and false indications in welds, 143
  mixed mode conversions, 18-19

modifier, 76, 77

molybdenum
  added to steel, 117

N

near field, 23, 47-48
near-surface discontinuities, 66
nickel
    added to steel, 117
noise, 101
non-consumable welding process, 132
noncontact ultrasonic techniques, 70
    methods compared, 71*table*
    transducers for, 58
nondestructive testing, 190. *See also* ultrasonic testing
nonmetallic inclusions
    castings, 119
    composites, 129, 130
    forgings, 128
    laminations in extruded rod and bar, 122
    laminations in plate and sheet, 120, 121
notches
    artificial discontinuities, special calibration blocks, 42
nuclear piping systems, 162
Nuclear Regulatory Commission guidelines, 178

O

oil
    as transducer couplant, 9, 62
on/off control, in pulse echo instruments, 32
on-site amplitude linearity checks, 102

P

paintbrush transducers, 51
partial penetration weld, 130, 131
penetration, 85
personnel certification, 7-8
personnel qualification, 5-7, 180
Personnel Qualification and Certification in
    Nondestructive Testing: *Recommended Practice*
    No. SNT-TC-1A, 5, 7, 181, 183, 189
petrochemical plant applications, 87, 147
phased arrays, 54
piezoelectric ceramics, 45, 46, 86
    use in through transmission technique, 65
piezoelectric effect, 45-46
piezoelectricity, 45, 76
piezoelectric materials, 45-46, 76, 86
pigs, for remote pipeline testing, 59
pipe (defect)
    castings, 119
    ingots, 117-118
pipelines

remote testing using pigs, 59
ultrasonic testing applications, 147
pipes
    angle beam testing, 92
    ASME standard, 182
    avoiding false indications, 162
    detecting discontinuities perpendicular to entry
        surface, 157, 158
    nuclear piping systems, 162
    production, 124-126
    shear wave technique application, 65
    surface wave technique application, 66
    ultrasonic testing applicable to, 4, 161
pipe welds, 124, 125, 162
    angle beam testing, 93
piping porosity, 128
plastics
    refraction by media, 21
    ultrasonic testing applicable to, 4
plastic wedges, mounting over crystal in contact testing,
    52, 53, 63
plates
    air coupled transducers for, 89
    angle beam testing, 92
    C-scan, 83
    detecting discontinuities perpendicular to entry
        surface, 157
    grid pattern scanning, 92
    high-speed scanning using bubbler technique, 68
    immersion testing, 90
    Lamb wave mode application for thin-walled, 14
    limited access tests, 165
    MIL-STD-2154, 186
    production, 120-121
    shear wave technique application, 65
    straight beam scan pattern on, 91
    surface wave technique application, 66
    ultrasonic testing applicable to, 4, 148
plate waves, 10, 11
plug mill, 124
plywood, 129
polarized ceramic, 46
porosity
    castings, 128, 129
    composite structures, 129, 130
    lenses, and distortion in beam profile, 175
    in welding, 139-140
welding processes associated with, 135
portable ultrasonic discontinuity tester, 25

ultrasonic testing for detection, 1, 75, 76, 147

W

water
    acoustical impedance, 16
    refraction by media, 21
    as transducer couplant, 9, 62
    use in contact testing, 62
    use in immersion testing, 62, 66, 67
waveform, 173
wavelength, 4, 5
    and sensitivity, 46
    and sound wave attenuation, 15
wear plates, mounting over crystal in contact testing, 45, 53, 63
weld discontinuities, 134-142
    false indications, 142-146
    perpendicular to entry surface, 157-159
    removed from entry surface, 159-160
welded pipe, 124, 125
weld groove, 131
welding, 125-126, 148
    ASME standard, 182
    ultrasonic testing applicable to, 8
welding processes, 132-134
weld joint configurations, 130, 131
weld root, 131
welds, 92-100, 130-132, 154-156
    detecting discontinuities parallel to entry surface, 149
    Lamb wave mode application for thin-walled plates and tubes, 14
    scattering discontinuities in, 160
    surface wave technique application, 66
    ultrasonic testing applicable to, 4, 130, 148
weld toe, 131
wetting agents, 62
wheel transducer technique, 67, 69-70
whiting, 4
wideband receivers, 170
wood products, air coupled transducers for, 89
worm-hole porosity, 128
wrought metals
    MIL-STD-2154, 186

Z

zero degree electromagnetic acoustic transducer, 59
zero offset control, in pulse echo instruments, 34